The Doctor's Book of Vitamin Therapy:

MEGAVITAMINS FOR HEALTII

The Doctor's Book

MEGAVITAMINS

by Dr. HAROLD ROSENBERG

Past-President, International Academy
of Preventive Medicine

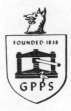

# of Vitamin Therapy:

FOR HEALTH

and A. N. FELDZAMEN, PhD

Formerly Editorial Director
of the Encyclopaedia Britannica Educational Corporation

G. P. Putnam's Sons, New York

Copyright © 1974
By Dr. Harold Rosenberg and A. N. Feldzamen, PhD

All rights reserved. This book, or parts thereof, must not be reproduced in any form without permission. Published on the same day in Canada by Longman Canada Limited, Toronto.

SBN: 399-11350-9

Library of Congress Catalog Card Number: 73-93743

PRINTED IN THE UNITED STATES OF AMERICA

Contents

Foreword

Testimony submitted by Dr. Harold
Rosenberg to the U.S. Senate Select Committee
on Nutrition and Human Needs

December, 1972

My practice is devoted to preventive care, the holistic concern of health of an individual through chemical analysis, nutrition, and exercise.

We need not be blind to reality. We are an affluent nation, but we are also malnutritious.

As a nation, we have a poor concept of what constitutes good nutrition. We thrive on excess carbohydrates and rely on our taste buds and visual sensations for sustenance. In most instances, we have not learned to eat to live, but rather to live to eat, and take for granted that what we eat is nutritious. . . .

Do we eat balanced meals? I categorically state we do not, and, furthermore, concepts of balanced meals do not necessarily fulfill the demands of cellular vitality. We are all biologically or biochemically individualized, and a diet for all does not necessarily satisfy all.

As a nation, we have little concept of the value of protein to our well-being. Nor do we have an iota of an idea as to the value of vitamins. . . . A house built of straw cannot stand under stress as well as one built of brick. A house based on protein needs protein. Vitamins are not freely available in so-called balanced diets. Frozen foods, packaged meals, are devoid of good nutrition. Meals missed, as

7

breakfast, and reliance on coffee breaks are poor substitutes for nutrition. Dietary fads based on single meals also contribute to poor health. Failure to eat soundly leads to poor physical performance as well as poor mental function and handicaps us socially and economically. Our total performance as a nation is retarded. Vitamins cannot be measured by minimal or recommended daily requirements. Some need more than others, and I feel RDA's [Recommended Daily Allowances] are inadequate. Vitamins are enzymatic in activity and, consequently, essential to our life's processes. . . .

There has to be a complete turnabout in our concepts. Our food industries, our advertising agencies, our educators, and our legislators must not take food for granted. . . .

It is not possible to indicate the importance of health care through nutrition in this short writing. I, as a practicing physician involved in preventive care and as past-president of the International Academy of Preventive Medicine, am optimistic about the future, but saddened by so much misinformation. We as a nation must not only indicate to our populace the right direction, but set the example for all nations. Preventive care means good health. Preventive care can only come through good nutrition, exercise, and understanding the biochemical rights of individuals.

CHAPTER 1:

New Vitamin Regimens for Improved Health

Let us be direct, frank, and to the point.

The purpose of this book is to allow you, the reader, to improve your health by means of a vitamin regimen, plus certain simple related nutritional practices.

Later in the book you will find these vitamin regimens, based on age, weight, height, and sex. They are to guide you, preferably with the advice of your physician, toward new and important steps to good health.

These new vitamin regimens are planned programs to increase vigor and longevity, reduce depression and fatigue, overcome anxiety and irritability, build up the body's defenses against disease, and help ward off actual illness.

Personal medical practice with dozens and dozens of patients has demonstrated the value of such high-level vitamin intake beyond any dispute.

Among those benefited have been many who thought of themselves as basically healthy. They did not always feel superbly fit, but when they visited a physician, the doctor could find nothing truly wrong with them other than a minor illness of the moment. They had no pronounced disease or serious chronic complaints.

Yet they were not getting all the vitamins they needed for full health and vigor. Nor enough protein. They were more tired, less vital, more liable to minor mental failings and illnesses than they should have been.

Often there were certain insidious symptoms, such as the inability to function under the slightest stress, forgetfulness, depression, and highly emotional states.

A health-building vitamin and protein program brought about improvement in nearly every case, sometimes dramatically and vividly.

Then there were other patients who had definite minor complaints, but these conditions were often difficult for them to describe. Years ago most physicians would have thought these symptoms impossible to diagnose or treat, calling them "neurotic" or "hypochondriacal" disorders. "Uncaused" heart palpitations, general debility and listlessness, for example. People often said these sufferers are "in poor health," without knowing why.

Many of such sickly and downcast types have also been given new strength and a sense of well-being by vitamin therapy.

This emphasis on nutrition and vitamins was not the start of this author's own medical practice, which for many years followed more standard lines. This practice included work in obstetrics, with the delivery of many babies. It included surgery. It included—and still does, when necessary—treatment for illness with medicinal drugs in the ordinary professional fashion.

But, in the course of time, it became clear that this was not the best health care for most patients. Treating people after they have become sick is a backwards approach. It puts the cart before the horse, because health, not disease, should be the major concern of medicine. It almost guarantees that we will have a high incidence of disease.

And all too often this treatment after-the-fact, called critical care, is ineffective because it comes too late. Although this "critical care" is essential when a person's health has significantly degenerated, we believe that greater health can be established and maintained by constant vigilance and attention to *preventive* measures taken before the patient gets sick.

One of the most productive preventive techniques is the application of a planned program of vitamin supplements.

New Vitamin Findings

Of course you have heard of vitamins. Everybody has. They are part of the general knowledge of our time, and there are countless newspaper articles, books, and even television commercials about them.

You probably know that each of us—man, woman, and child—needs vitamins in the diet to maintain good health. This means that vitamins are a *necessary food.*

But Dr. Robert S. Goodhart, writing in *Postgraduate Medicine,* notes that: "Many people subsist on diets that are inadequate in vitamin content to meet their requirements. To protect them against the development of vitamin deficiencies, it is necessary to resort to the use of supplemental vitamin therapy."

Perhaps, if you are in your middle years, you can recall your mother giving you cod-liver oil when you were an infant, because it had "vitamins." If you are younger, it is more likely that you were given vitamins in pill form as a child. In fact, you may take vitamin pills now, perhaps irregularly or even every morning, with juice. They can't hurt, most people think, or they might do some good. Why not?

If you are older, vitamins may have come to your attention during your own lifetime. The theoretical existence of vitamins only became known some years before World War I, in the second decade of this century. And it took decades after that for scientists and doctors to discover the individual vitamins themselves, to learn of their chemical and physiological properties, and to begin to understand their relationship to human health and disease.

Fewer than fifty years ago, for example, pellagra was still

a mysterious, wasting disease that afflicted many in the United States, especially in the South. People died of pellagra by the hundreds. Nobody knew it was caused by a nutritional deficiency or that a simple change in diet would provide the vitamin needed to eliminate this dreaded malady.

Vitamin research, of course, is still going on. New experiments and studies continue to add to our knowledge. Vitamin research is far from being a closed and finished chapter in medicine; recent discoveries actually show that we may be just at the early pages of the long vitamin story.

For example, the antistress properties of vitamin C and *pantothenic acid* (a B vitamin), and other vitamins, are now being investigated, as are the protective powers of many vitamins against cancer.

There is evidence that several vitamins have the power to lower the cholesterol circulating in the bloodstream, and this may be significantly related to heart and circulatory diseases.

Severe mental disorders have been a mystery to medicine from the beginnings of civilization up to the present day. But now there is new hope for such puzzling maladies as schizophrenia and childhood autism—via the new vitamin methods and related nutritional treatment.

These are recent medical and scientific discoveries. They come from laboratories, clinics, hospitals, and doctors' offices, all over the world. Altogether, they have given a tremendous boost to our hopes for better health and greater longevity for millions of people.

What Is a Vitamin?

There are three distinguishing characteristics that entitle a substance to be called a vitamin.

First, a vitamin is a naturally occurring "organic" compound, which means it is a chemical substance not found raw in the earth like a mineral, but must (in the natural state) be created by living things, by plants or animals.

Of course pure vitamins can now often be manufactured in the laboratory as well or on a larger scale for commercial purposes. But, even in the manufacturing process, living organisms are often used, similar to the way we "manufacture" beer, wine, yogurt, certain cheeses, honey, etc.—using other organisms to do our work for us.

Second is the fact that a vitamin is a necessary food for growth, good health, or reproduction. In fact, if our diet is deficient in vitamins, we become much more prone to illness. Physical damage will become evident, and this is often accompanied by mental disturbances as well. The mental signs of vitamin lack may precede the physical symptoms, and may range from the very mild to the most severe.

The insufficiency or absence of a vitamin may take many weeks, or months, or even years to become noticeable. Or the effects of a deficiency can be relatively rapid. A long-continued lack of such a necessary substance can lead eventually to serious disease or disability, and then possibly to death.

How is this known? In some cases, by studies of human disease, such as the mortal deficiency diseases of scurvy, beriberi, and pellagra. In other cases, by animal investigations in which the experimental animals are fed deficient diets and the results carefully observed. The researcher then attempts to relate the findings to the case of man.

In short, the human body cannot manufacture the vitamins it needs from other foods, yet it cannot live in health without them. This is how vitamins are defined, and why they are termed "essential in human nutrition."

The *third* touchstone as to whether a substance is a vitamin is the *quantity* required by the body. Compared with other foods, vitamins are needed in only minuscule amounts. The average adult eats about 3.5 pounds of moist food daily. All the vitamins combined that are needed to avoid any obvious signs of vitamin deficiency come to less than 1/300 of an ounce each day. Even the new high-level vitamin regimens use very small amounts of vitamins, against the scale of our customary intake of proteins, fats, and carbohydrates.

Thus the vitamin concept is that certain organic compounds are necessary in tiny quantities for good health. This is now accepted without question and seems obvious and natural. But this concept did not exist before the turn of the century. Medical science of that time was absorbed by the then-recent discovery that germs or microbes could cause human disease, which was itself an epochal step forward in the history of medicine.

Vitamin knowledge came later. Largely, this knowledge was gained by observations of health disorders in man and animals. These health disorders result from deficiencies. Even today, the focus of vitamin thinking is often on disease and infirmities. We would prefer to turn our attention to health instead because good health rather than the absence of illness should be the goal of medicine and its related arts.

The Need for Vitamin Supplements

It is often said that if you eat the proper foods and have always done so, then you have probably gotten sufficient vitamins for the needs of your mind and your body.

"On the other hand," Professor Jean Mayer (former Special Consultant to the President on nutrition) tells us, "If your food habits are irregular, if for one reason or another there are certain classes of food that you have been directed by your physician to omit, if there is, in short, any reason to suspect the adequacy of your vitamin supply, then you will be advised [by your physician] to take vitamins."

The general belief had been that only certain tiny

amounts of vitamins are needed for the best health, just a bit more than the minimal amounts that prevent the obvious signs of deficiency. But the new vitamin discoveries, especially in the past half dozen years, have caused many physicians, scientists, and other concerned specialists to alter their thinking.

Now it seems more and more clear that far larger quantities of vitamins are often desirable for many people. It is being demonstrated that up to ten, a hundred, or even a thousand times more of some vitamins are often beneficial.

Dr. Leon Rosenberg (no relation) of Yale University has reported on nearly a dozen metabolic disorders that have been discovered—all since 1954—that impair the body's utilization of vitamins to such an extent that a person may require hundreds of times the so-called minimum requirement.

Dr. Bernard Rimland, a San Diego psychiatrist at the Institute for Child Behavior Research, notes: "There is an extraordinary amount of prejudice against the idea that a vitamin—a perfectly safe naturally occurring chemical that we all require to sustain life—can be required by some people in large quantities. Every physician has heard of Vitamin-D-resistant rickets. While most children need only 400 units of Vitamin D to prevent rickets, others need up to 500 times as much."

And Professor Linus Pauling, Nobel prize-winning biochemist and a leader in vitamin research, states clearly: "*Probably almost everyone would benefit by supplementing his ordinary foods by the especially important foods called vitamins. . . . If we lived entirely on raw, fresh plant foods, as our ancestors did some millions of years ago, there would be no need for concern about getting adequate amounts of the essential foods, such as the vitamins. The vitamin content of foods is decreased by modern methods of processing and also by cooking. Accordingly, it is often necessary to supplement the diet by ingesting additional amounts of these important foods. . . .*"

Dr. Robert S. Goodhart: "It must be emphasized that supplemental vitamin therapy is a means of protecting the individual against the development of vitamin deficiency states and is a means of maintaining normal tissue reserves against the demands of unusual stress situations, such as illness, injury and pregnancy." And he notes further: "Disease and injury may increase vitamin requirements, interfere with their ingestion, absorption or utilization or increase elimination. . . ."

Knowledgeable nutritionists such as Linda Clark, Dr. Carlton Fredericks, and others, whose primary emphasis is generally on a good diet of nourishing natural foods, today also urge additional vitamin supplementation. Such nutritionists report that they carefully and extensively augment their own diets with vitamin supplements, and often they recommend this for others.

Why? One gave her reasons: "Anyone who has been ill or whose previous diet has been inadequate needs much larger quantities [than the "minimal allowances"] of nutrients except calories. . . . It is doubtful whether these allowances are actually sufficient to maintain health; certainly they are inadequate for any person whose health is below par . . . supplements should be continued as long as the nutrients they furnish are not being obtained from any other source."

Benefits of the New Vitamin Regimens

No evidence from others or theoretical reasoning is as strong as what one sees himself, repeated over and over, with patient after patient.

What does vitamin therapy do?

The best way to describe the result is to call it *an improvement in health.* No longer are faces so drawn and anxious or bodies weakly slumped. There is a new outlook of vigor and a change in the totality of consciousness—the patient often seems visibly to "brighten." He or she will report an enhanced performance, physical and mental, in everyday life.

The new keenness and vitality can be obvious. Optimism and self-confidence have replaced a negative viewpoint. Inexplicable downcast feelings are cast aside. Where there was fatigue and weakness, now there can be stamina and strength. And minor illness and complaints, such as colds and miscellaneous aches and pains, are no longer as troublesome as they used to be.

Simple, safe, and relatively inexpensive, such vitamin therapy, coupled with other forms of good nutrition, has especially marked effects with many over 35 years of age. The new bodily and mental strength often leads to a higher degree of physical activity, including healthful exercise, which now becomes *pleasurable* for many who cringed at the thought of physical exertion before.

Sex life? A vigorous interest in sex is a sign of good health. In both men and women this should continue throughout adult life, even into the eighties and nineties, with performance to match this interest.

Many patients, both men and women, have had their sex lives recharged with vitamin therapy.

Are you a person with run-of-the-mill health? Is your weight far from what it should be, over or under? Do you feel less vital, more depressed and anxious, than you used to be? Do you have outbursts of temper, followed by self-recriminations that make you feel as though you would just like to crawl into a hole and lie there?

Do you shun many activities because you "don't feel well," claiming that you are rundown and tired? Do you look back for comfort to your successes of the past, rather than looking ahead for new challenges and triumphs?

Do you think that your current state of health, physical and mental, is the best that can be expected?

If so, then the chances are high that you are mistaken

—that a proper vitamin regimen could well improve your *bodily metabolism* and *mental functioning* to a noticeable extent.

You yourself know that there are times when you do feel truly well, full of energy and vitality, self-confident, at your peak. This should be most of the time, not just once in a while.

Could improved nutrition, primarily via a vitamin regimen, help bring you to such a peak more often as a normal state of affairs?

We do believe that additional vitamins, properly administered, are likely to bring such benefits to you now. Furthermore, they may add substantially to your longevity.

As we have noted, the primary basis for this claim is personal medical practice, but we can happily report that many other physicians and scientists are also noting surprising benefits from the new vitamin regimens. In some cases it is a relief of distressing symptoms; in other cases it is an increased feeling of well-being; in still others there have been laboratory findings of gains in longevity, growth, or reproductive capacity among animals. Even intelligence and mental alertness have been shown to be improved among humans and animals by high vitamin intake, demonstrating the value to the mind, as well as the body, of the necessary foods we call vitamins.

Since we are recommending vitamin supplementation so strongly in this book, one other point needs to be mentioned very clearly. No one associated with this book—not the authors, editors, or publisher—has any financial interest, direct or indirect, in any vitamin product or company.

Thus this book is not "advertising" for vitamins. It *is* a recommendation for good health practices for the reader.

Causes of Success of the New Vitamin Regimens

Nobody can fully explain the success achieved with so many patients by the new methods of vitamin therapy.

Perhaps for some individuals vitamin treatments counteract the aftereffects of poor nutrition in the past. As we shall see, it is likely that all of us have suffered malnutrition earlier in our lives. In fact, Dr. Daniel T. Quigley, author of *The National Malnutrition*, claims: "Everyone who has in the past eaten sugar, white flour or canned food has some deficiency disease, the extent of the disease depending on the percentage of such deficient food in the diet."

And George L. Mehren when he was Assistant Secretary of Agriculture pointed out that a survey by his department showed that "18 percent of households do not fully meet approved intake of one or more nutrients."

Also, it is known that some people are born with distinctive personal vitamin needs, far above the average. The "typical" individual is a medical fiction who does not truly exist. Each of us is a unique person, born with a personalized body chemistry unlike that of any other human being.

The doctrine of "biochemical individuality," proposed by Professor Roger J. Williams, the distinguished biochemist and one of the nation's leading experts on nutrition and disease, means that everybody is likely to have some vitamin needs far above the average, even at birth.

Then, as infancy and childhood life progress, these specialized needs may become accentuated. Years of poor nutrition or dietary indiscretions as an adult can also affect our body chemistry, further altering the "optimum," or best, quantity of vitamin intake for each of us.

Another proposed explanation is that we have all along been underestimating the most desirable quantities of vitamins for maximum health for most people. Many are still alive who were born before the first vitamins were discovered, so medicine and science have not yet had the time to study and investigate vitamin needs fully, especially as related to long-term effects.

Vitamin knowledge is so new that the probable finding of a new vitamin, provisionally named vitamin Q, was just announced in late 1973 by Dr. Armand J. Quick and his colleagues in Wisconsin. It also just came to be known that high intakes of *folic acid* (an often neglected B vitamin) may prove important in countering the damage inside our arteries that may have arisen from drinking homogenized milk. And a new 1974 report from Glostrup Hospital in Denmark indicates that vitamin D therapy "definitely reduced" the number of seizures among hospitalized epileptic patients, all of whom had been receiving anticonvulsant drugs for years.

Unfortunately, our government agencies have not been providing timely leadership in the field of vitamins, often lagging behind scientific knowledge by many years, with possibly serious consequences to our total national public health. It was as late as 1968, for example, that the Food and Nutrition Board officially listed a "Recommended Dietary Allowance" for *pyridoxine* (vitamin B6), though the importance of this vitamin had long been known. And while more than 8,000 medical and scientific research papers about vitamin E have been published in the last twenty years, the Food and Drug Administration did not include this vitamin in its list up to 1973, so that the most widely used vitamin supplements entirely omitted this essential nutrient well into 1974.

And a major public and scientific controversy about the merits of vitamin C *(ascorbic acid)* in preventing or alleviating the common cold has yet to be fully settled. Surprising new research from Canada, which we will describe later, has apparently resolved some of the hotly debated questions, but it has raised other, equally puzzling ones for investigators to ponder.

Add to this the fact that vitamins are needed in small amounts, and it will be understandable why many believe we may not yet have discovered all the vitamins. There are "vitaminlike" substances whose status is still in dispute.

Dr. Morton S. Biskind, writing in the *American Journal of Digestive Diseases*, tells us: "Several misconceptions . . . have become increasingly prevalent. One common misconception is that all the important nutritional elements have already been isolated and indeed, that a number of those currently available are not significant in human nutrition. . . ."

So not only are the optimal quantities of the known vitamins still in question, but also the full array of necessary nutritional elements.

One other important proposed explanation for the success of the new vitamin regimens must be mentioned. This is the hypothesis that modern conditions of living have raised our needs for supplemental vitamins.

Recent years have seen a great increase in excessively processed and refined foods without nutritive value. When these fill the diet, they crowd out more nutritious foods and contribute to cellular deficiencies. The hazards of white flour, refined sugar, and high-heat "solvent-extracted" vegetable oils, which together bulk large in the American diet, have not been fully explored. These provide "naked calories," without the other food elements necessary to metabolize them, and they drain the body of vitamins and minerals.

Highly processed and refined foods—convenience foods and special snacks, artificial drinks, imitation juices and so-called fruit "-ades" and packaged dinners—all contribute to the need for extra vitamins, as do many drugs.

Americans now consume 4,000,000 pounds of artificial colors each year, twenty times more than in 1940. Many such dyes once widely eaten are now banned because they produce cancer in laboratory animals.

Another distressing aspect of modern life is the presence of pollutants and other environmental poisons that we unavoidably ingest and breathe. An ever-increasing barrage of new chemicals reaches our bodies through food and water consumed, air breathed, and drugs taken. Vitamins are known to play an important role in helping the body rid itself, when it can, of such deleterious foreign substances, which are agents of environmental stress.

Further, many believe that we now live under conditions of exceptional personal or social stress. Ours is a time of "future shock," it is said, whereas former generations led more settled and placid lives. Then there was more ease and contentment. Now changes seem to occur overnight. New technologies, changes in political affairs, unsettled personal living and marriage conditions, career and work uncertainties—all cause stress. And here again, several vitamins are known to be related to stress, especially certain B vitamins and vitamin C.

One knowledgeable commentator, for example, describing her own use of vitamin supplements, noted that vitamin C requirements climb "if you're under stress, if you smoke or eat stuff with poison sprays or chemical fertilizers in it, or if you breathe smog. Most of us couldn't *hold* enough fruit, tomatoes and cabbage to supply our needs these days."

Steps Toward Better Health for You

The aim of this book is to provide you, the reader, with clear and specific broad-spectrum vitamin regimens to benefit your health.

We believe such a vitamin regimen is likely to bring you a renewed vigor and sense of well-being that you may not have experienced for many years.

But should you begin a high-level vitamin regimen and, with it, a protein diet, the benefits may not be apparent the next day or even in the first week. None of the changes occur overnight. Several weeks are sometimes required before the results can be strongly felt. In some cases, several months pass before the full effects come on, and a year or longer may be necessary to reverse certain internal chemical patterns completely.

As we shall see, this may be because new internal tissues may have to be formed, and such growth takes time. So patience will be necessary.

Many books about vitamins and nutrition intended for

the public have been published in the past few years, stimulated by the new discoveries. Some of these are measured and calm works, written with a clear intent of objectivity. Others are almost hysterical, implying that the medical profession has been blind or corrupt in not recognizing the value of vitamins. Often the stress is on disease—as is frequently inevitable in vitamin writings because the value of such nutrients is usually measured by researchers against various states of ill health—but these writers go further.

They often leave the misleading impression that many or most human illnesses or infirmities can be "cured" by vitamins. This is unfortunate because it is scientific folly. Such a false impression can lead a misinformed reader, who has only been given a collection of half-truths, seriously astray, especially if he unwisely attempts to doctor himself for a health complaint.

Self-medication, without skilled diagnosis and laboratory testing procedures, is a foolish activity, and it can be a dangerous one.

Any reader who suspects he is sick or who has a troublesome health complaint should get professional care from a physician or dentist.

Similarly, because each of us has an individual chemistry and a unique style of life, we hope that your own vitamin program will be adopted under the guidance of a physician.

Let's tell the truth. Not all doctors believe in the efficacy of vitamin regimens. Nutrition, as we shall see, is not much taught in medical schools. The large pharmaceutical companies invest *thousands of dollars a year per physician* to persuade them to use drugs. The government agencies tell us repeatedly that we are a well-fed people and have no nutritional failings. Many of the important vitamin discoveries have taken place only in the last decade. So it is to be expected that a majority of doctors should not be knowledgeable about vitamin therapy.

But happily, more and more physicians are coming

to know about the beneficial effects of vitamin regimens and wholesome food, since the evidence of their health importance is mounting up each year. Later in this book we will describe much of this evidence and some of the theories that have been advanced to explain the powerful biomedical effects of vitamins.

But what about your own vitamin program, if you are not clinically ill? In the ideal case, you will find a physician who is grounded in the principles of nutrition, who knows your medical history and can monitor your bodily changes as you take the vitamins. Ideally, too, he (or she) will have a holistic concern for all aspects of his patients, their health as well as their diseases, and understand the importance of preventive medicine, as well as that of critical care devoted to disease.

Indeed—let us be very clear about this point—the treatment of health complaints should never be do-it-yourself medicine but should have the best professional care.

But the *prevention* of illness by good health habits, including proper nutrition (which in our world today means vitamins), does lie in the sphere of the layman as well as the doctor, and possibly even more so. Who would not rather prevent a health disorder than try to cure one?

Maintaining and improving health by vitamins and diet are the goals of this book. We have written it because so many have had an unexpected new fitness and vitality result from a systematic vitamin regimen. They have turned into new people, as they have said, with a mental and physical vigor and feelings of well-being that they had forgotten all about—after many past years of droopy fatigue and covert depression.

We hope that you may be among those who will gain from vitamin therapy. We hope that you too can have the benefits of all the vitality, strength, and alertness—all the vigorous good health—that you should have.

CHAPTER 2:

The Fallacies of the "Balanced Diet"

One newspaper account tells of a flagpole sitter who flourished on his lofty perch for many weeks on a diet of biscuits, algae tea (a nourishing brew), and ordinary tea. Another newspaper story tells of two young men cast adrift on the ocean who survived seventy-two days each on one cup of seawater and a tablespoon of peanut butter daily, and one cup of rainwater and a half can of sardines every five days.

The human organism has such enormous reserves of chemical strength to combat temporary emergencies. Over the long run, however, when time is measured in years and decades, even these reserves can be worn away. Nutrition has major long-term effects for good or ill that profoundly affect our health and longevity.

For decades, nutritionists have been attempting to formulate simple rules by which we would all be assured of receiving nutritious foods over the long term. To do this, they have often divided foods into groups. At one time there were as many as nine groups. The current fashion is to speak of only four food groups:

- Meats (including fish and poultry)
- Milk and dairy products
- Fruits, and yellow and green vegetables
- Cereals and grains

25

The idea is that a person eating some of each group daily—or in each meal—will be assured of being well nourished. This would constitute the "balanced diet" that is supposed to be desirable.

Of course, it is always possible to choose nonnutritious foods from each of the four groups and so end up by being badly nourished. This is one flaw or fallacy in the concept.

Another fallacy is that people's distinctive personal needs for nutrients vary so greatly among different individuals that merely "balancing" different types of foods, like adjusting a fuel mixture for a gasoline engine, cannot hope to cover the variations. Different people are not like similar engines. One person may be placid, relaxed, easygoing, while another is active, tense, seemingly under strain, always fidgety and in motion. A single balanced mixture will not serve to meet the needs of such different types of metabolisms and functionings.

The "food group" thinking has also been questioned by those who have special dietary inclinations. Vegetarians, for example, wish to discard the meat group and often the dairy group as well. Others claim that man can live nutritiously on meat and fish alone—and indeed he probably can if many parts now ordinarily discarded are included in the diet, especially if raw. The word *Eskimo* in fact means "eater of raw meat," and their former raw animal and fish diet in a bygone age did contain many vitamins now destroyed in cooking—Vitamin C, pyridoxine, etc.

Animals and the Balanced Diet

On a purely scientific basis also, the "balanced diet" concept does not stand up. In fact, some have pointed out that few animals in their natural state eat a balanced diet. How, then, do they get the vitamins and minerals they need?

Dr. Henry A. Schroeder and his associates at the Dartmouth Medical School and Brattleboro Memorial Hospital have pondered this question, especially as it applies to minerals, which are similar to vitamins. They note: "From the viewpoint of the evolutionary dietary history of the human race, it is logical to believe that every major natural source of caloric energy carries with it the inorganic nutrients necessary for its metabolism. This statement holds for all animals; otherwise deficiencies would occur and species would either become extinct or would have to depend on more than one source of food for survival (i.e., a 'balanced' diet)." The same is true for vitamins.

These researchers state they know of no wild animal on land or sea that requires a "balanced" diet. Modern man and his domestic and laboratory animals may need such diets because pastures are overcropped or otherwise depleted of trace elements and foods are prepared from many sources and processed in ways that destroy their original nutrients.

Dealing with the case of *pyridoxine*, vitamin B6, for example, which is destroyed by the heat of cooking, the Texas physician Dr. John M. Ellis is skeptical that modern civilized man can ever receive enough from his ordinary food. "Unfortunately, it is probable that during the lifetime of every person living today, supplements will be necessary, for there are few, if any, Americans, certainly, who have received the optimum daily intake of B6 from fetal life to the present. Supplementation is the only way left in which to overcome what is probably some degree of deficiency as a result of our having eaten food that is either overcooked, overprocessed, or to some extent depleted or devoid of B6."

Similar remarks could be made about other vitamins. No possible "balanced" diet, even of the best natural and wholesome foods, is likely to meet all our nutritional needs today. *Thus the main theoretical fallacy is that a balanced diet eliminates the need for vitamin and mineral supplementation.* This erroneous idea is often repeated, especially by those who are unaware of the newer thinking and research findings about the value of vitamin and mineral supplementation.

Even the prestigious Food and Nutrition Board of the National Research Council and the generally antivitamin Food and Drug Administration now reluctantly agree that some trace nutrient supplementation (iron) is necessary for "normally healthy" individuals because ordinary food is insufficient.

Further, as we will see, our age of biochemical civil war against ourselves and of prepared and processed foods —foods that are neither fish nor fowl, neither wholesome plant product nor simple dairy one—places many everyday food choices outside the scope of any four or seven or even nine basic food groups and makes even a good diet difficult for many.

The Need for Vitamins

Saying that a "balanced" diet does not fully meet all our nutritional needs today is not the same as saying that ordinary food is unimportant. But merely selecting from the basic food groups is no cure-all for malnutrition or related metabolic defects owing to bad eating habits, fad diets, drugs (such as pep and diet pills, barbiturates, alcohol, etc.), foods raised on mineral-depleted soils, pollutants and contaminants, or heavily processed artificial foods.

In place of the "balanced" diet concept, we might be better off were nutrition education to stress a *varied diet of natural and wholesome foods, plus adequate trace nutrient (vitamin and mineral) supplementation.* Put another way, the "balanced" diet idea is acceptable *if it includes the needed vitamin and mineral supplements.*

Dr. Neil Solomon of the Johns Hopkins Medical School notes:

Since the discovery of vitamins, particularly in the 1920's and 1930's, there was a great furor and hoopla about the necessity for adequate vitamin consumption since many diseases, such as pellagra, beriberi, rickets, etc., were found to be caused by lack of vitamins in the human diet. In the days and years that followed the early research into the properties and values of various vitamins, widespread publicity in the lay press was given to the importance of these vital elements of the daily diet.

Since the general popularity of the fad diet has infused our overweight society, it would appear that most of what the public learned and took seriously a generation ago has become watered down in many minds. Nevertheless, the fact remains that vitamins are an integral part of any balanced diet, some vitamins obviously playing a more important role than others.

Dr. Solomon goes on to stress his belief that laymen should not decide their own vitamin intake, but should have their supplementation under the guidance of a knowledgeable physician, which, of course, is the best way.

A recent survey of patients in the large hospitals of a major city showed that more than half had deficiencies in either vitamins, minerals, or protein, and many were deficient in more than one of these categories. Most of these patients probably believed they had been eating a "balanced diet." Let us bear this in mind as we take a brief—if frightening—glance at our national public health.

CHAPTER 3:

The Decline of
Public Health

Anyone who examines our national pulse is led to many questions about nutrition in general and the American diet in particular. Are we a well-fed people? If so, why is our life expectancy so low, compared to other nations? The United States ranks eighteenth in the world in male life expectancy, according to the latest figures, just a hairbreadth above the Soviet Union. Among the nations ahead of us are Italy, Hungary, and Greece, so it is not just the small-population, highly prosperous, socially calm Scandinavian countries where, on the average, a man will outlive an American.

This is a shocking finding. Almost equally distressing is the fact that we rank fourteenth or worse in infant mortality. Did you know that a baby born in Japan or France has a greater chance of survival than one born in the United States?

These are *comparative* results, relating public health in the United States to that in other nations. But there are also *absolute* measures of declining public health, such as the rate of low-birth-weight babies. A "low-birth-weight" baby is a full-term infant that weighs less than five and a half pounds. This sign of malnutrition correlates directly with mental retardation, cerebral palsy, and a host of other permanently damaging birth defects. It is an unhappy fact that the number of low-birth-weight babies has gone *up* in the United States by 143 percent from 1960 to the present.

Also, hypertension (high blood pressure) is going *up*, in the sense that more and more people are getting it, but also going *down,* in the sense that it is appearing at younger and younger ages.

Further, as another indication of absolute decline, this time in mental health, not only do we have a continuing or increasing high suicide rate, but the murder rate has *doubled* in the United States in the decade from 1962 to 1972. This situation is grim: In 1972 there was a 5 percent increase over 1971 in the number of murders per 100,000 people.

Other indications of our poor public health abound:

- For females, our ranking in life expectancy is only eleventh in the world.
- A male American of 20 will have a shorter total life span than his counterpart in 36 other countries.
- An American woman 20 years old will be outlived by her counterparts in 21 other countries.
- A 40-year-old male American can expect to live only 4.1 years longer now, than he would have in 1900, despite all the benefits of modern "critical" medicine and health care.
- Among 17 industrial nations, the United States ranks second in one important statistic for males aged 40 to 50. This statistic is the death rate. The United States has the second highest death rate during these productive years among all these nations.

Perhaps you are thinking that this distressing mortality record is due exclusively to the poor in our society. Yes, the poor do drag the figures down, but this is not the whole story. It doesn't ·fully explain the prevalence of chronic and degenerative diseases among the well-to-do and affluent.

Is it that we do not have enough competent doctors or hospital beds? We do know the training in critical medicine of our health professionals is among the most rigorous and best in the world. And we also know that the number of physicians and hospital beds have kept pace with the growth of the population. There are 45 percent more working doctors now than there were in 1950, for example, so a lack of physicians is not behind our health troubles.

In fact, health care is the third largest "industry" in the United States, employing nearly 4,000,000 persons and costing some $70 billion annually, nearly 8 percent of our gross national product.

Indeed, we have twice as many surgeons per capita as Great Britain, and each of our surgeons performs as many operations as the British surgeons. The rate of operations was 7,440 per 100,000 population in the United States in one recent year, and 3,770 per 100,000 in Great Britain. Yet Great Britain is tenth in the world in male life expectancy, far outranking the United States!

What is it that is killing us so tragically and so prematurely? Heart and circulatory diseases (including strokes) account for more than half our national deaths. If cancer is added in, the total then comes to more than 70 percent.

These afflictions that bring death are called "mortal" diseases, and they can be preceded by "premortal" signs, which can range from high blood pressure, ulcers, and neurological conditions to extreme disabling conditions.

Mortality is not the only area where, as Ralph Nader's Study Group reported in 1970, "statistics support the picture of deteriorated American health." Experts also look at "morbidity," which means chronic or disabling illness. Here our record is also a sorry one. For example, 11 percent of our population have "chronic conditions causing activity limitation," according to a recent study. *This is to say that one American in ten is to some degree an invalid.* Heart conditions, rheumatism, and arthritis cause nearly one-third of such activity limitation, and none of this appears directly in the longevity statistics.

When we pause to reflect on these matters, we are often inclined just to shrug our shoulders uncomprehendingly and utter a few generalizations about the overly rich American diet or the "stress" in modern life.

Stress and Malnutrition

There are two kinds of stress in medical thinking. One type is called *personal* or *social*. This results from "active" life-styles, individual career or family pressures, frustrations, resentments, lack of sleep, and so on.

Other stress is due to the *environment*—extremes of heat and cold, drugs and chemicals, pollutants, noise, radioactivity, and other external factors.

It is believed that stress of both types is significantly related to many of our health shortcomings. The importance of stress in medicine is attested to by the existence of a special professional journal devoted to it because stress is known to cause many bodily (and mental) changes.

The ability to withstand stress is often a direct function of nutrition. This is known from hundreds of experiments dealing with deleterious chemicals, energy expenditures, bacterial and viral infections, studies of irritability and depression, hormones and enzyme levels, and so on.

*Mal*nutrition means "bad" nutrition, not merely undernourishment. Stress and malnutrition together are believed to be the major culprits in our sad state of health.

Have we actually become a malnourished nation?

Dr. Stanley N. Gershoff of the Harvard School of Public Health recently reported that a survey of nutrition studies conducted between 1950 and 1968 showed that the American diet has deteriorated, *especially since 1960*. A significant portion of the population is now receiving less than half of the recommended daily allowances of vitamins.

Biochemical measurements in the "deficient" range are widespread.

This is particularly important because many of the people studied were not impoverished but of the middle class. Dr. Gershoff noted that *"nutrient inadequacies are not confined to the poor or the old, but reach into all income groups and all regions."*

Dr. Grace A. Goldsmith is dean of the School of Public Health and Tropical Medicine at Tulane. In 1972 she testified in Congress about the major "Ten-State Nutrition Survey" that had been reported that year.

This large-scale survey showed that "a significant portion of the population surveyed is malnourished. . . . Many children and adolescents *in all population groups* are underweight and short in stature. . . . Obesity is common, particularly among adult women. . . . A high prevalence of *low* hemoglobin and hematocrit [red blood cell mass] values was found in *all segments of the population.* Poor dental health was encountered frequently. Many pregnant and lactating women maintain low serum albumin levels, suggesting marginal protein nutrition. Low levels of vitamin A are common and riboflavin [vitamin B_2] status is poor. . . ." [Emphasis added.]

And Ralph Nader's Study Group Report, *The Chemical Feast: Report on the Food and Drug Administration* by James S. Turner, laments that the Food and Drug Administration will not acknowledge the relationship between deteriorating American health and the limited availability of safe and wholesome food.

"In fact, American food consumption patterns play an important role in the nation's disgracefully high infant mortality rate, low rise in life expectancy, and seemingly insoluble problems of stroke, heart disease, and cancer."

The relationship between nutrition (including vitamins) and the health of our public has spawned an almost unprecedented amount of public controversy, and given rise to wholly new and bizarre life-styles among our younger people. We now have back-to-nature communes all across the land. Health food shops have become a commonplace. Newspapers and magazines are filled with articles about food, nutrition, and pollution. Fad diet books make the best-seller lists, a new one each year. Government agencies and Congressmen are deluged with mail when changes in the vitamin and mineral regulations are proposed.

The public apparently, as never before, is concerned with nutrition because people everywhere are uneasy about their health. This fact itself is often mentioned as a sign that something is wrong on a national scale with our nourishment and the environment.

CHAPTER **4**:

The Decline of
Nutritional Food

Before the turn of the century, people ate nutritious wheat products made from stone-ground flour, and they often sweetened their food with natural honey and crude maple sugar. Vegetable oils (even made by simple pressing at normal temperatures) were a rarity. Vitamin-rich fresh fruits and vegetables were eaten soon after harvest or not at all, for there were few ways to store and maintain fresh produce.

Many lived close to the land, on farms or in nearby small towns, and except for cereal grains and home-preserved fruit, plant products usually had to be eaten in season. Pork, rather than beef, was the chief animal food, and animal fats were the mainstay for frying, baking, and other kitchen uses.

Our ancestors, though they had their diseases, were a hearty, strong, self-reliant, and cheerful people.

White Flour, Refined Sugar, and Extracted Oils

The first major change in the food supply was the introduction of steel-roller equipment to mill wheat, our basic grain foodstuff. The "efficient" new rollers, which became commonplace about 1910, could grind the wheat kernels very finely, removing most of that perishable part called the wheat "germ" and allowing only the starchy compo-

37

nent to remain. After bleaching and further processing, the result was an ultra-refined white flour, nearly pure starch, that soon became standard.

Today we know this process removes at least 22 *known essential nutrients*, including most of the entire B-complex of vitamins, vitamin E, important oils and protein amino acids, and necessary minerals such as calcium, phosphorus, potassium, and magnesium.

Millers and bakers, however, liked the new flour. If kept dry, it could last for indefinite periods without spoiling. ("Spoiling," by bacteria, molds, fungi, or insects, means that these other living organisms find the food sufficiently nutritious to satisfy their appetites and support their life processes.) "Instead of being alarmed by the decreased nutritive value of white flour as shown by the inability of insect pests to thrive on it, the production of white flour was hailed as a great forward step," wryly noted Professor Samuel Lipkovsky of the Agriculture College of the University of California at Berkeley.

White flour is our basic grain foodstuff. Not only bread, but also rolls, cakes, pies, cookies, doughnuts, pancakes, waffles, spaghetti and other pasta products, gravies, breadings, pastries, pizza, and many other foods are made from it. But our modern bleached and refined white flour is so low in nutritive value, as Gary and Steve Null point out in their informative book *The Complete Handbook of Nutrition,* that "even insects shy away from this product—showing marked preference for the whole grain bread and cereals."

About thirty five years ago, just prior to World War II, millions of our young men were examined by their draft boards. Officials were distressed to find a large fraction physically or mentally unfit for military service. Alarmed by the poor state of our national health, the government began a mandatory "enrichment" program for flour used in bread, in which at first three and later four important nutrients were restored: the (inexpensive) vitamins thiamin, riboflavin, and niacin (vitamins B_1, B_2, and B_3), and the mineral iron. Little attention was paid to the other missing nutrients, some of which, in fact, were unknown at the time, nor to other uses of flour (cake, pies, etc.). The enrichment program has remained essentially the same to the present day.

During this century, Americans were also developing a sweet tooth—a penchant for sugared foods that would grow until, at present, we would each on the average be consuming more than two pounds of sugar each week. Raw types of sugar are particularly susceptible to spoilage, so sugar refining was soon able to produce from cane or beets an ultra-refined foodstuff, more than 99.9 percent pure sucrose. Because of the dangers of microbial contamination, it was made unlawful to sell any sugar less refined. Today all apparently partly refined sugars, such as brown sugar and "Kleenraw" (a fancy crystalline type often found in smart restaurants), are actually made by adding molasses to refined white sugar.

Removed of all the vitamins and minerals required for its metabolism within the body, this sugar began to find its way in ever-increasing quantities into a host of both traditional foods (cakes, pies, pastries, candies) and newer "convenience" foods (breakfast cereals, soft drinks, fruit "ades," chewing gum, frozen and canned goods, imitation meals, and so on).

One result was an extraordinary amount of tooth decay. Dr. Abraham Nizel of the School of Dental Medicine at Tufts wrote in 1973 about the effects of dietary sugar on a once-primitive people, the inhabitants of Tristan da Cunha:

In 1938, the diet of the natives consisted of two staples, potatoes and fish but no sugar. Not a single first permanent carious molar was found in any of the young people under the age of 20. In 1962, they were consuming an average of one pound of sugar per week, per person, with the result that a comparable age group showed 50 percent of their molars to be carious.

Vegetable oils were the third high-energy (that is, high-calorie) food to become important in "modern" times. These oils are made from nuts, grains, beans, seeds, and olives. The old method of manufacture was simply to squeeze these in a press until the oil came out, but only two materials, sesame seeds and olives, yield enough oil this way for modern standards without heating them first. (Only such oils can truly be called cold-pressed.)

A second method uses a screw press (like a corkscrew): Cooked material, usually at temperatures between 200 and 250 degrees, is thereby squeezed until the oil is forced out, producing "expeller-pressed" oils (though fraudulent organic or health food merchants have sometimes misleadingly called these cold-pressed also).

"Solvent extraction" is the major commercial method for extracting vegetable oils today: This is a high-heat process in which the ground-up materials are cooked with steam and mixed with a petroleum solvent and then heated further to remove the solvent. Then the oil is refined with caustic lye (at temperatures around 450 degrees) to remove impurities, and further bleached, filtered, and deodorized. The result is a colorless, light, bland oil, almost tasteless. Often the oil is then "hydrogenated" to make it more solid for use in margarines, peanut butter, baked goods, and other foods.

The "impurities" that are largely removed by such severe processing include the "health food" lecithin (which contains phosphorus and the important B vitamins choline and inositol), "essential fatty acids" that are necessary in human nutrition, and fat-soluble vitamins, such as vitamins A and E.

Flour, sugar, and oil are three basic foodstuffs, the starting materials for many cooked or processed foods. But the modern methods of manufacturing them have produced devitalized "foodless" foods, stripped of nearly all nutrition except calories. There is good evidence that (even if "enriched") they rob the body of B vitamins, disrupt calcium and other mineral metabolism, cause obesity and overweight, contribute to circulatory disorders, and have a damaging effect on the nervous system.

For example, Professor Roger J. Williams in Texas performed a revealing experiment with the assistance of Charles W. Bode some years ago. They used 128 weanling rats. Half of the animals were given commercially enriched bread as food; the other half got the same diet, but with added supplements of vitamins, minerals and one protein amino acid.

Ninety days later two-thirds of the test animals in the first group had perished of malnutrition, and the remaining third was severely stunted. Those in the second group, which had received the supplements, were mostly alive and well, with growth and development seven times greater than the surviving deprived animals.

Another experiment, done more recently in England, focused on white refined sugar. The able Dr. John Yudkin informs us that rats that had been flourishing on an ordinary diet were switched to a diet identical in all respects, except the starch calories of the former diet were replaced by sugar. In short order, diabetes and circulatory complications developed.

"Modern" Food Technology Arises

As these three ultra-refined foods were coming into prominence during the past half-century, other important changes were also under way in agriculture and food processing. What were once small family farms gave way to large agricultural combines. Small food handling and manufacturing companies became giant industrial corporations. And Americans got to want and demand many fresh food items on an all-year-round basis.

Robert Choate, chairman of the Council on Children, Media, and Merchandising, caused a national furor in 1970 when he testified in Congress about the nutritional damage done to children by most breakfast cereals. Later, in 1972, he testified again about how World War II was a turning point in nutrition and food merchandising.

> Prior to World War II, old town or old country knowledge of the food supply was handed down through generations from grandmother to mother to child. Whether it was shelling peas, scrubbing potatoes, rolling pie crust or cleaning fish, the child of that generation picked up food knowledge by helping in the kitchen.
>
> During the years prior to World War II, typical meals in the United States had identifiable ingredients or came from recipes proven through decades and centuries to be capable of sustaining some degree of nutritional health. Prior to World War II, many citizens of the United States were still producing some of their own food supply and hence paid attention to the quality of the eggs produced by their own chickens or to the color of the carrots produced by their own vegetable gardens.
>
> The military requirements of World War II produced a host of food technology innovations. Meals for our armed forces had to stand storage for months. Snacks called K and C rations became substitute meals. Drinks from powdered ingredients and eggs and milk in a dry-pack cardboard box came to be common. Cartons and their liners were studied to resist insects, rodents, and mildew. . . .

After the war, armed with this new technology and buoyed by an expanding population and exceptional prosperity, the food companies began to develop variations on old foods at a fantastic rate. Choate went on to note: "Processed foods, using basically inexpensive materials that were coaxed into supposedly fascinating new shapes, colors, and smells, came to be advertised and glorified out of proportion to their nutritional contribution. Processed foods with heavy advertising could afford a higher mark-up, which justified further advertising. Basically nutritionally-worthwhile items such as fruits, vegetables, inexpensive cuts of meat, and low cost legumes rich in vegetable protein disappeared from television advertising as major dollars were put behind the contrived foods . . ."

Food advertising rose 4 times from 1955 to 1970, from $181 million to $683 million. The products most advertised were (and are) the least nutritious: desserts, condiments, fats and oils, starches, snacks, and so on.

The Expansion of Food Processing

Today the food industries are in total the largest retail business in the United States, an enormous and increasingly concentrated industrial complex. For example, two producers dominate the soft drink industry, with only four other major competitors. Most of the breakfast cereals—85 percent—are made by only four companies. The dairy industry is tightly organized on a regional basis. Major meat packers are parts of financial conglomerates, as are baking and milling companies. Most of our canned and frozen goods are also produced by only a handful of companies. Two companies sell more than half of American cheese; two companies sell most of the salad dressing; *one* company sells 95 percent of all prepared soups.

The five largest food-processing companies are truly industrial giants, each with sales over $1 billion. The leader, Beatrice Foods, does nearly $3 billion in business each year, making it nearly as large, all by itself, as the entire broadcast television industry. The General Foods Corporation is number two, with annual sales of about $2.6 billion, and with 430 different food products, including Birds Eye, Jello, Kool-Aid, Maxwell House, Sanka, Yuban, Maxim, and the Burger Chef and Rix food chains. Such companies have larger receipts than the Gross National Product of many nations. One food retailer, in fact, has 2,300 super-markets in five different countries.

General Mills, another top five processor, is also one of the large breakfast cereal manufacturers. But it makes other products as well. In 1972, for example, agents of the Food and Drug Administration seized General Mills' butter pecan cake mix. It contained neither butter nor pecans. Instead it had date bits and artificial flavors. But the law was insufficiently powerful to make the seizure stick. The same cake mix is still being marketed with neither pecans nor butter, while the FDA stated it would be seeking stronger legislation to give it the power to deal with such abuses!

Such supercorporations must obey the laws of the marketplace and financial community, if not the intent of our governmental laws. In particular, there is constant stockholder pressure on them for greater earnings and increased sales. Profits and growth are always the stern measures of success in our business economy. But these goals have become increasingly difficult in recent years because our population growth has slowed (to a tiny 2 percent annually) and most Americans are eating less food than before (due to less physical effort expended in ordinary activities). But how can these companies try to achieve growth and earnings?

One answer is to sell services as well as food. This means more and more processing of raw foods. The company not the housewife now peels the potato—and it also minces, flakes, dehydrates, steams, boils, bakes, fries, and cans, boxes, and freezes it. Sometimes the result, when finally prepared to be eaten, is a product that bears a similarity to a familiar food, such as mashed or fried potatoes or potato chips, even if it is made in a wholly new way. Food chemists can now often break a raw food down and then rearrange or reconstitute it, producing what the Food and Drug Administration, almost at a loss for words, has just decided to call "restructured foods." Fried clams, fish sticks, potato chips, dairy products (so-called filled milk, in which vegetable oils replace the butterfat), and so on.

Another answer to the search for profits by the super corporation is to produce wholly new foods, such as snack and convenience items (pop tarts, breakfast squares, instant meals, etc.), of which about 1,000 new types are tried by the marketers each year. Much more emphasis is placed on advertising and packaging than on nutrition, but, luckily, most of these ersatz "foods" fail to gain public acceptance. But in the process of their trial, the housewife is bewildered by having to choose among the approximately 10,000 items in the average supermarket, and millions do eat such terrible junk.

As the new food products come to the store shelves at a record clip, their "life cycles" have dwindled from two or three years in the mid-1960's, to six months or less today. Nobody can keep up with so many new foods—not nutritionists, government agencies, or ordinary citizens.

One commercial disadvantage to such heavily processed foods is the high cost of labor, and labor costs often go up and up as more services are applied to raw foods. In fact, workers who processed and sold food last year collected nearly as much in wages as all the earnings of all the farmers who grew all our crops and raised all our livestock.

So another answer to the need for increasing profits is to use *cheaper ingredients*. As consumer protest movements against high prices have grown and raw food costs have risen, more and more companies have taken this route. Harvard nutrition professor Jean Mayer points this out clearly:

> The net effect of this pressure on the food industry —increased costs and the consumer resistance—is that, like all other industries, they are going to look for cheaper and cheaper sources of raw materials. The cheapest sources of raw materials are *sugar and hydrogenated vegetable fat.* Modern food technology enables you to make

foods that look like other foods even though they are made differently. I believe that unless we react to what has happened, we will end up with a debased food supply. [Emphasis added.]

Even some of the finest restaurants have succumbed to such modern food technology, often serving (at the highest prices) frozen steaks or roasts that have been precooked and frozen and then are warmed in microwave ovens for serving. Once common only in the quick-service food chains, this is fast becoming the practice in the luxury trade as well, and for the most expensive dishes: rack of lamb, lobster, pompano, and so on. One person who applied for a position as a chef was told cooks were no longer needed, only "thawer-outers."

Serving temperature remains a problem in these restaurants. Precooked meats in roasts cannot be served both hot and rare (because extended recooking would bring them up to medium or well done), so they must be drenched with heated gravies or sauces. For turkey or duck this is expected, but the customer who orders his rack of lamb rare and unadorned is likely to find cold meat on his heated plate. The "homemade" loaves of bread on many restaurant tables are another example; these are made from frozen dough, and the New York *Times* calls them "fairly sad nourishment."

Synthetic or frozen juices, frozen fish, nondairy "cream," and similar artificialities are now also becoming the rule rather than the exception. After a few drinks, customers can only rarely tell the difference between artificial or precooked frozen foods and old-style cooking, and while the new foods are more costly, unserved portions can be kept and labor costs reduced.

One fictional chronicler of our modern malaise is the gifted writer John Cheever, who wrote: "They ate frozen meat, frozen fried potatoes, and frozen peas. Blindfolded one could not have identified the peas, and the only flavor the potatoes had was the flavor of soap. It was the monotonous fare of the besieged . . . but . . . where was the enemy?"

Agribusiness

At the other end of the food supply, on the land, important changes have also been occurring in the last decades. Agriculture became big business. No longer do we grow food for our own use and send machine-made products abroad—our "agribusiness" today actually furnishes a dollar majority of American exports to the rest of the world. The United States is now the world's largest exporter of wheat, soybeans, and even rice.

American know-how turned easily to improving our agricultural production in the twentieth century because big profits were at stake here too. We learned how to fertilize our land to produce hitherto unknown high yields of grain, vegetables, fruit, and fiber. We learned how to breed plants for better growth, and also how to breed livestock and artificially fatten them (with sex hormones), and so increase our yields of all animal products as well.

As our own—and the world—population grew, we found ever more powerful ways to kill bacteria, fungi, weeds, molds, insects, and animal pests that threatened a food supply that had to grow to match. Business methods—and business thinking—were applied on the farm (now sometimes even owned by a canner or other food processor), as well as in the factory.

The new technology also catered to the desires of Americans for fresh produce all year long. Fruits and vegetables came to be harvested earlier and earlier, before they were ripe (and before achieving their full quota of vitamins and minerals), and then artifically "ripened" with ethylene gas. After that, they were often waxed to give them an inviting appearance and to avoid spoilage owing to water losses by evaporation. Oranges, lemons, other citrus fruits, apples, melons, cucumbers, new potatoes, and other produce are thus routinely chemically ripened and coated with wax today.

In addition, fruits and vegetables may be stored for long periods at low temperatures under "controlled atmosphere" conditions—that is, surrounded by inert gases to retard visible spoilage. (This is now commonplace in the handling of apples, pears, cherries, strawberries, and other fruits.) Antisprouting chemicals that inhibit growth are applied to fresh root vegetables, such as potatoes, and other chemicals are used where the color is an important factor.

Our Tasteless Foods

Other historical factors also affected our attitudes toward food. Jet aircraft travel and low-cost student fares to Europe permitted tens of thousands of young people of moderate means to take a "grand tour" abroad, beginning in the late 1950's. The results would have been predicted.

These young people, less influenced by television, tasted the foods of other countries as yet unaffected by the new food technologies, and returned to the United States and our own often dreadful table fare. In revulsion, they spurred into national prominence the health food and back-to-nature commune movements.

In a different way, older Americans who were also traveling abroad in greater numbers, also reacted against the poor quality of domestic food. But we did this by a heightened interest in "gourmet" cooking, in taking wines with meals, and by a growing and sometimes amusing snobbery about restaurants.

Young and old have been seeking good nutrition, but this search has masqueraded as a quest for deliciousness.

Much of the current interest in food—the cookbook craze, the popularity of the TV cooking shows, the step-up in wine on the American table—stems from a vast, unrealized striving for nutritious health-building foods. It is the biochemical wisdom of our bodies expressing discontent with nonnutritious, processed, warped, and degraded foods.

The human tongue is an extraordinarily acute "chemoreceptor"—which means it has very delicate sensing mechanisms. Our sense of smell is even more acute. Together, the tastebuds of the tongue and the olfactory receptors in the nasal passages make up the sense of taste, which is very responsive to trace elements—more so, in many cases, than the laboratory chemist with all his apparatus.

Europeans and other foreigners who come to our shores have often remarked on the tastelessness of our food, especially the flatness of the "fresh" fruits and vegetables, and Americans abroad are often startled by their first bites of truly fresh and tasty foods. This greater tastiness is due to healthful nutrients, to which we are naturally chemically responsive. The tastelessness of our domestic foods means less nutritive value. The lack of taste may also have other health consequences.

More than half of all adult men and 40 percent of the women in the United States are more than 10 percent overweight today. About one-third of the men are actually more than 20 percent overweight. Obesity is thus a national epidemic, with major damaging health consequences.

This excess weight comes from overeating. We do not do the heavy physical work our ancestors were accustomed to, and now we need fewer calories. Total caloric intake has dropped, but not enough to make up for the difference: we still tend to eat far more than we should. Some have proposed that this overeating on a national scale is due to a lack of genuine tastiness in our domestic foods. The body, actually seeking nutrition, may be impelling us to eat more and more, and so to excess.

Further, such tastelessness may be an important factor leading to an excessive use of salt, spices, and other condiments. We pour these on our foods in an effort to restore flavor in our mouths, and here also the results are considered by many experts to be damaging on a mass scale to our health.

The American housewife herself is partly responsible for the tastelessness of our foods. She usually chooses to buy by appearance, rather than for flavor or nutrition. When buying fresh fruit or vegetables, for example, she looks first for size, color, and firmness, believing these are the signs of quality. Those in the business of supplying food must cater to our buying habits—and we have rightly been called a nation of nutritional illiterates.

Nutrition vs. Profit

Recently a new variety of tomato, called Carored, was developed at Purdue University. This has ten times the vitamin A content of conventional varieties, but also an orange-red color. Food marketers felt this unusual color would lead to consumer rejection of the Carored tomato in spite of its significantly improved nutritional value, and so it never came to market.

Mr. Edwin A. Crosby directs the Agriculture Division of the National Canners Association, a commercial trade organization. He recently observed: "At the present time, Purdue University is considering the introduction of a new tomato variety having a brighter red color than present varieties, but interestingly enough, having approximately half the Vitamin A content of most present day varieties." By such steps, little by little, have we seen the decline in our national nutrition and the loss of vitamins.

The business of farming must also impel the growers of plant crops and those who raise livestock to seek profits and to select the varieties of plants and animals that will lead to marketplace success.

In the case of plant foods, a high yield per acre is most desirable when choosing among different strains. The plants to be raised should grow bountifully, have an early maturation, high levels of resistance to disease and insect pests, and be adaptable to a wide range of weather and soil conditions. Also, growth to a uniform size and the ripening of separate plants at the same time are desirable so the plants can be harvested at one time by machines or migrant workers.

If the crop is to be sold to the public as fresh produce, then its weight and appearance are also important. *Flavor is distinctly secondary, and nutrition hardly enters the question.* Fruit, for example, that is colorful, juicy, plump and firm will always bring the highest prices; more flavorful and nutritious fruit, but less appetizing in appearance, goes to the bottom of the barrel.

One of the controversies currently exciting consumer groups, government agencies, and food growers and processors is *nutritional labeling.* The proposal has been made that all foods—boxed, canned, and frozen foods, fresh produce—be labeled with their content of protein, carbohydrates, fats, water, vitamins, and minerals. Leading the opposition to this are the food growers and many commercial canners. Mr. Crosby spoke about this, and his reasons are interesting.

"Let us now look at why fruits and vegetables are included in the American diet. It would seem there are two basic reasons, one nutritional and the other esthetic. From the standpoint of pure nutrition, principal consideration in fresh fruits and vegetables should dwell in the area of vitamin content, and secondarily, mineral content. It is to be questioned, however, whether the average housewife thinks nutrition when she buys these crops or whether she isn't more concerned about variety, color, esthetics, flavor, texture and other factors in her menu planning than total nutrition.

"If we move to nutritional labeling, then we may well have a large number of consumers awakened to the realization that fruits and vegetables are *not* generally good sources of nutrients from an economic viewpoint, and if she is truly concerned about insuring that her family receives enough vitamins and minerals, the easy economical route to insure this end is to purchase them in pill form."

Of course, one reason that fruit and vegetables in America are not good sources of trace nutrients is that they have been bred and raised to meet other criteria. Another is that even were the growers to try to improve the nutritional qualities of our foods, the public might reject their efforts unless it was better informed.

Further, there would be an inevitable time lag, especially for apples and other such fruits grown on trees, before any upgrading of nutritional value could ever be achieved by plant breeding, even were the growers to attempt it. Trees take years to grow. "Any substantive change in the varietal picture of tree fruits could hardly be accomplished in this century," according to Mr. Crosby.

Nutritional labeling and more nutritious crops are desirable goals, however long range. But in the meantime, one must agree with one of Mr. Crosby's points: Vitamin supplements are the only sensible way to insure adequate nutrients in the diet today.

CHAPTER 5:

Vitamins Are Also Foods

This may be one of the most important concepts in nutrition. Vitamins are not drugs or peculiar stimulants or alien chemicals—vitamins are *foods*.

But despite their presence in many other foods, vitamins can be fragile compounds, readily destroyed or removed by many common or even necessary practices.

Some of these vitamin losses are inevitable because the heat of cooking, soaking in water, exposure to steam, the action of air on cut or chopped foods, storage, freezing, antagonistic food additives or pollutants, and even light, can each destroy vitamins. When peas are soaked in water for only ten minutes, for example, they lose 20 to 40 percent of their *thiamin* (vitamin B$_1$) and 35 percent of their vitamin C. The B vitamins and vitamin C, all water soluble, are readily left behind in the cooking pot water, especially when vegetables are overcooked or steamed for a long period. Moist heat is damaging: potatoes containing 40 mg of vitamin C when raw have only 4 mg, one-tenth as much, when cooked and reheated for serving.

The dry heat of toasting destroys *pantothenic acid*, an important B vitamin, in breads and other grain foods. Baking soda also destroys many of the B vitamins. The heat of pasteurization, aeration, and light destroy vitamin C in milk: One writer believes we lose more vitamin C each year by the pasteurization of milk than is contained in our

53

entire citrus crop. Potatoes stored for three months, even under good storage conditions, can lose half of their vitamin C content. Freezing and storage for long periods destroy vitamin E.

In the days when the milkman left his goods in clear bottles on doorsteps, the early morning sunlight would destroy the *riboflavin* (vitamin B2). Now when milk is irradiated to produce vitamin D, this light also cuts the riboflavin content.

Often antagonistic elements in foods reduce the amount of vitamins the body can absorb. Raw egg white destroys the B vitamin *biotin*. Rancidity in fats and iron salts destroys vitamin E. (Unless bile and fats are present in the intestinal tract, the fat-soluble vitamins A and E cannot be absorbed.)

Vitamin D is believed to be produced *on* the skin, not within it, by the action of sunlight. If one washes immediately before and after sunning himself, the vitamin D-producing oils are washed away. Without the presence of calcium, ingested vitamin D cannot be absorbed.

Although carrots are widely thought to be a good source of the material carotene from which the body can manufacture vitamin A, this carotene is within the indigestible vegetable cell walls. If the carrots are raw and not chewed thoroughly, as little as 1 percent of the carotene may be available to the body. Cooking breaks down these cell walls and does not injure vitamin A, so cooked carrots may provide 5 percent to 20 percent of their carotene to the body.

Mineral oil, which has no food value, can flush the four fat-soluble vitamins A, D, E, and K from the body. Antihistamines and sulfa drugs destroy vitamin C and the B vitamin *PABA*. Aspirin and barbiturates also destroy vitamins, and antibiotics that injure the intestinal flora cut down on the vitamin K and the B vitamins that these friendly bacteria can produce. Smoking lowers the level of vitamin C in the blood.

Malabsorption in the digestive tract can prevent vitamins from being used by the body. Insufficient hydrochloric acid in the stomach or weak digestive enzymes, often found among older people, can impede the absorption of B vitamins and vitamin C, and insufficient bile or the absence of necessary minerals hinders the absorption of fat-soluble vitamins.

But food processing and cooking are the chief vitamin thieves. For example, up to 98 percent of the vitamin E is lost in the process that makes cornflakes, and 90 percent in the ordinary milling of wheat. In making rice cereal products, the loss is about 70 percent. The B vitamin *niacin* (vitamin B3) is also lost.

There are often also substantial seasonal variations in the vitamin contents of both vegetable and animal foods. There can be an eightfold difference in the vitamin E in cow's milk, from 0.2 International Units (IU's) per quart in the early spring to 1.6 IU's in the fall. Winter butter and eggs usually contain far less natural vitamin A than the summer products.

Where and how crops are grown and harvested, or animals foraged, are also important to their vitamin content. Early harvesting of immature plants leads to vitamin-reduced produce. Fertilizers are important: The level of thiamin in grain crops has been doubled by good use of the proper nitrogen, potash, and superphosphate fertilizers. When certain plants were grown on soils fertilized with animal manures only, the carotene (provitamin A) contents were substantially less than when appropriate chemical fertilizers were added.

The mineral content of foods is even more susceptible to soil conditions, especially if "organic" or "natural" farming methods are used. If a soil is deficient in a certain mineral, then manures from local animals or composts from decaying vegetation of the region cannot provide the needed minerals, since these minerals cannot be created by any living things. *"Organic" farming methods can thus perpetuate a local soil deficiency rather than correct it.*

Modern life habits—often also unavoidable—frequently

drain vitamin resources. For example, long exposure to harsh and glaring lights is a commonplace among office workers. This uses up vitamin A at an accelerated rate, with consequences of increased susceptibility to colds and minor infections, complexion problems, and night blindness.

Alcohol, which is a special "pure" carbohydrate, increases the body's needs for vitamins, just as white sugar and white flour do. Thiamin, pantothenic acid, niacin, and other B vitamins are depleted in alcoholism, as is vitamin C. Food additives and pollutants, which we will deal with in the next chapter, are also injurious to the vitamins in foods, as well as in our bodies.

Is this not a dreary catalog of nutritional woes?

Most of the public is vaguely aware of the body's needs for additional vitamins. A recent survey by the Opinion Research Corporation in 2,000 interviews used the question: "Do you think there is *a definite need, some need,* or *little or no need* to have vitamins added to food products?"

Over 70 percent responded that there was *a definite* or *some need* for additional vitamin fortification, and 86 percent of those between 18 and 29 years felt this way.

But people are unaware how many vitamins are needed and how much. And they do not know how to get these vitamins in their diet of ordinary foods or which supplements to take.

Both food growers and processors have been sensitive to these feelings, seeking greater public acceptance and sales of their products. More and more the food processors add vitamins to their foods, especially to children's breakfast cereals. They advertise "8 IMPORTANT VITAMINS" or "10 ESSENTIAL VITAMINS" to attract the public, using the least expensive and incomplete collections of vitamins.

Too many food companies have indiscriminately begun "to spray vitamins on whatever they happen to make," notes microbiologist Michael Jacobson, co-director of the nonprofit Center for Science in the Public Interest. This center recently published his 102-page booklet, *Nutrition Scoreboard*, in 1973, which rates food on a point system —adding points for protein, naturally occurring carbohydrates, vitamins A, B_1, B_2, B_3, B_6, and C, iron and calcium and trace minerals, while detracting points for added sugar and saturated fats. (This useful booklet is available at $2.50 from The Center for Science in the Public Interest, 1779 Church Street N.W., Washington, D.C. 20036.)

Noting that these fortified products are often nutritionally equivalent to vitamin-coated candy, it cites a popular cupcake which is not nutritious, despite the added vitamins, with a low score of minus 44 on the "nutrition scoreboard."

Such foods must also be assigned to the "un-natural" category, to be avoided by all who seek better health. Dr. Jean Mayer again: "Enrichment has always been partial . . . a diet high in white flour, hydrogenated vegetable fat and sugar—even if enriched with a comprehensive list of nutrients—would still be a harmful diet. . . ."

CHAPTER 6:

Vitamins and Pollution:
Our Biochemical Civil War

A high standard of living, but a low quality of life.

Nobody need be told that we have too often disrupted the delicate balances of nature for the sake of material progress, and then seen the results boomerang against us. We all know the environment is polluted. But few are aware of the effects of this chemical warfare that we have been waging against the environment—that it has also been against (and within) ourselves, truly a civil war in which we have attacked our own bodies.

Contamination in the air, water, and land is increasing all over the world, and among domestic and wild animals and plants as well. Sickness and injury rise as this contamination invades our tissues. The effects have been hastened in the United States by our advanced technology and the many branches of science that industry has fostered for its own purposes.

Air Pollution

Air for breathing is a prime requirement of human life: Each of us must breathe about 15 times a minute, night and day, as long as we live, taking about 30 lbs. of air into our bodies each day.

But into the atmosphere over the United States we have been releasing each year some *200,000,000 tons* of serious

59

pollutants, about one ton per person. More than half come from our gasoline vehicles; the rest from factories, power plants, municipal dumps, and private incinerators. Journalists have rightly called many of these pollutants "unseen enemies," for many are gases that are *invisible* and *odorless*. Others are tiny particles of solid matter—tars, poisonous heavy metals (lead, beryllium, etc.), and other damaging substances, sometimes so fine that a single breath may contain 70,000 such solid particles—yet 80 tons of such heavy dust falls on each square mile of Manhattan each month.

The gases include carbon monoxide, the sulfur oxides, nitrogen oxides, and ozone. These can sear the lungs, affect the oxygen-carrying capacity of the bloodstream, attack the eyes and respiratory passages, and leave us weakened and mentally foggy.

There are two types of damage from such air-borne poisons. First is the immediate and evident damage from brief exposures. These affect the elderly or chronically ill with special force, causing respiratory disorders, irritation of the eyes, nose, throat, and ears, and more seriously, worsening existing bronchitis, emphysema, asthma, and heart conditions. We have become so used to air pollution that we are no longer shocked when the local news announces a "pollution alert," and then calls off the grim statistics of increased hospital admissions and additional deaths.

The second type of effect, slow and insidious, is due to long-term exposure. Many authorities are now convinced such exposure *causes* lung cancer, stomach cancer, emphysema, bronchitis, a lowered resistance to respiratory infections and influenza, certain mental weaknesses, and many other disorders. Long-term effects are difficult to measure, but the evidence piles up. For example:

- Among English *nonsmokers*, a careful study showed a tenfold difference between the death rates for lung cancer in rural and urban areas. A person breathing polluted metropolitan air often inhales as much benzopyrene (a known cancer-inducing hydrocarbon) as he or she would by smoking two packs of cigarettes daily.

• The higher level of heart attacks in our cities is believed related to air pollution. Death rates from coronary heart disease are 37 percent higher for men and 46 percent higher for women in metropolitan areas with high atmospheric pollution levels than they are in nonmetropolitan areas. Cardiovascular death rates are more than 25 percent higher for male Chicagoans between 25 and 34 years of age than for their counterparts in rural areas, for example. The difference is 100 percent for men between 35 and 54, and nearly 200 percent for men between 55 and 64!

But even before the energy crisis caused a lowering of our clean air standards and a rise in air pollution, this inescapable hazard was reaching beyond our larger cities. One writer left Manhattan to return to Missoula, Montana, once called The Garden Spot of the West, but he could not escape the smog. "When I lived in Manhattan," he said, "I used to watch the clinkers come down the airshaft and remember how great the pine-scented evening downdrafts smelled in Missoula. . . . Today Missoula is the country's second worst smog area." Signs were posted on the highway by outraged citizens: MISSOULA, MONTANA—*DIRTY SKY COUNTRY*.

Lower grades of coal and oil will now be burned in power plants and factories to cope with the energy shortage, and our air will be increasingly fouled. Each individual will have a greater need for adequately nourished cells in the lungs and other respiratory passages, for such cells are more resistant to pollutants and have increased recuperative powers.

As we will see, vitamins play an important role in the body's "first-line" defense against such external irritants and hazards.

Water Pollution

Water is another of the prime necessities of life. Each of us takes in on the average about 2 lbs. of water daily; without water, survival beyond a few days is impossible.

But in addition to drinking our water, we have also made it a vehicle for the removal of human and industrial wastes and a drain for the chemical agents applied to our land. Our lakes and rivers have become great cesspools. Even the surrounding oceans are despoiled: Travelers in small boats on the Atlantic thousands of miles from shore have noted filth and trash floating by, evidence of the reach of our civilization.

And over 23,000,000 Americans are now drinking water that federal officials have called "potentially dangerous." More than 6,000 communities are involved. Water-borne epidemics of such bacterial and infectious diseases as cholera and typhoid fever seem to be increasing. In addition, the exotic new poisons emerging in ever-growing numbers from industrial plants and factories, falling from the sky and draining from the land, are believed to be causing thousands of other cases of water-borne illnesses each year.

The contaminants include fertilizers, herbicides, fungicides, insecticides, irrigation residues from agriculture, animal and human wastes, detergents from home and industry, radioactive wastes from power plants, industrial and research institutions, a spectrum of heavy toxic metals, a wide variety of chemical salts, and many other materials.

But nobody is certain as to the concentrations at which numerous contaminants, such as organic poisons and heavy metals, cause adverse health effects. Some of these effects are only identifiable after years of exposure, so the cause-and-effect relationship is not easily found.

Environmentalists also point to another danger from water-borne contaminants, not to ourselves but to our offspring. Many pollutants are believed to cause genetic changes, so their injurious effects can carry forth into future generations, affecting our children, the children of our children, and beyond.

Again we will find that vitamins are important, not only to nourish and strengthen the body's natural defense mechanisms, but also as actual poison-combating agents themselves.

Land Pollution

Our contamination of the environment is not only conducted in the air and water—it also takes place on land.

"When they first came in, I thought it was heat exhaustion," said Dr. Charles Keagy of Delano Hospital in California. Two farm workers in the citrus, grape, and cotton country had arrived for treatment.

"They were sort of in a state of exhaustion, perspiring heavily and vomiting. But it became obvious it was pesticides. They became incontinent of urine and feces—and their muscles were trembling. They had been spraying a parathion solution and the hose came loose and sprayed material on their pants."

"We don't see these severe cases too often," he went on. "Most of the time it's mild cases—just some muscle spasms and difficulty in breathing."

Parathion is one of the newer "organophosphate" pesticides, originally created for the military for chemical warfare, but now being increasingly used to replace the DDT that was banned in 1972. Such poisons attack the nervous system and inhibit necessary enzymes in the bloodstream. They are permitted to be used because unlike DDT, they are not long-lasting, but decompose after several weeks. Nevertheless, studies show they are getting into our food supply.

One drop of pure parathion on the skin can cause convulsions, coma, and death. A 7-year-old boy strolled through a field that had been sprayed shortly before with this pesticide poison—and fell dead almost immediately. In a more bizarre case, parathion continued to work after death, sickening both the doctor and coroner who were handling the body of a parathion victim.

Some of the minor symptoms have often been taken for those of influenza—nausea, vomiting, dizziness, headaches, heavy sweating, cramps, and general malaise. Only expensive laboratory tests, rarely performed, can distinguish such minor pesticide poisonings from influenza.

More severe pesticide poisonings can produce uncontrolled ulcerations of the skin with pus-filled sores, bloody urine, and muscle spasms in the esophagus. Victims suffer from intractable bleeding from the mouth, nose, and eyes, and then respiratory arrest leading to death.

Parathion is only one of many virulent poisons used in agriculture. Aldrin, dieldrin, guthion, ethion, nicotine, lead arsenate, methoxychlordane, benzene hexachloride, lindane, are some of the others, equally powerful. One half teaspoon of dieldrin is fatal to man, and 16 farm workers were disabled with sickness after entering a field treated two full weeks earlier with ethion.

Altogether there are in use on our farms about 1,000 such highly toxic agents in 32,000 different commercial products—all to kill bacteria, insects, weeds, fungi, molds, or animal pests.

The Environmental Protection Agency officially recorded nearly 6,000 severe pesticide poisonings in 1970, before the usage of the organophosphates increased. But an official of the Food and Drug Administration felt the true number had been unreported; his own estimate was 80,000 pesticide poisonings a year, and 800 or more deaths.

There is no question that some of the greatest advances in human health and well-being have been owing to such pesticides. They have spectacularly improved the food supply all over the world. They have helped reduce much disease and sickness. It is impossible to say how many hundreds of thousands or millions of people have had the opportunity to live out their life span, rather than die, probably at an early age, of malaria, typhus, or some other insect-borne disease.

But in terms of other factors, many of these pesticides have been a mixed blessing. By its powerful effects on mosquitoes, DDT virtually eliminated the major killer, malaria, in many areas and minimized its effect in others. But in 1958 Dr. Malcolm M. Hargraves of the Mayo Clinic testified in court that he was certain DDT also caused leukemia, aplastic anemia, Hodgkin's disease, jaundice, and other fatal blood disorders in man.

DDT, like many other poisons, can accumulate in the body, slowly building its concentration to dangerous levels, though there is evidence that vitamin A affords some protection against its effects. After many years of argument and soul searching, DDT was banned in the United States in 1972—though its residues remain in all our bodies. The mite-killer Aramite was also found to be a slow cancer-producer and eventually also banned, but not until after it too had been used extensively.

Cumulative, irreversible, slowly damaging our health, pesticides have come under increasing attack by concerned civic and medical groups. The Yearbook of the *American Journal of Public Health* has noted that "contrary to previous beliefs, it now seems likely that a substance which is poisonous to one form of life is very apt to be found to some degree toxic for other animals, includ ng men."

Chemical fertilizers are another mixed blessing. Without them, our crops would not reach their bountiful growth, we would not have an adequate food supply, and the nutritive value of many crops would be lowered.

But again, there are no gains in dealing with the environment without some problems. Many fertilizers or their components, if not removed from our food and water, are a hazard to human health. The mineral cadmium, for example, an ingredient in certain fertilizers, has been shown to be implicated in the kidney complications of persons suffering from extreme high blood pressure, and animal experiments have duplicated this finding.

Just as vitamin A has been shown to be a valuable agent against DDT, so vitamin C is protective against this toxic mineral cadmium, as well as against other deleterious fertilizer residues. Some of these residues are nitrogen compounds, nitrates and nitrites, which even appear in the milk from cows that drink water polluted by fertilizer drainage. Infants are particularly susceptible to such chemicals because they have not yet developed certain metabolic enzymes; in fact, the effect of nitrates on infants is a blood disease which leads to death if intake is not stopped. Older children and adults have higher immediate tolerances for these nitrogen compounds, but there is evidence that within the body, they are turned into dangerous cancer-producing substances, nitrosamines. Interestingly, here too the latest evidence indicates that protection—if it can be provided at all—is most likely to come from vitamin C.

Animal Pollution

Our domestic animals are fed on grains and grasses, and they drink the local water, so they ingest all of the chemical agents with which we treat the land and plants, and which we discharge into the waters and skies.

In addition, strong poisons, antibiotics, sex hormones, and even tranquilizers have been and are widely used to increase livestock growth or productivity. Cattle, poultry, hogs, and sheep are routinely treated this way—these agents being placed in their food, used as a skin dip, or implanted in their bodies.

Arsenic is routinely used in chicken feed today. Antibiotics and tranquilizers serve the same purposes for animals as they do for humans, to prevent or overcome disease, and to keep the animals placid, contented. "Milk from contented cows" used to be a heavily advertised slogan. One doesn't see this anymore, perhaps because the company fears consumers will think the cows have been "tranquilized" and refuse to buy the product.

But when tranquilizers do increase milk or egg yields, keep animals from unnecessary self-injury, or enable them to mate more readily, you can be sure that unless forbidden, they will be extensively used.

Much attention has gone to sex hormones, expecially diethylstilbestrol, DES. This is an artificial female sex hormone, once used widely to fatten poultry and cattle, and also used medically in women to control threatened abortion or heavy bleeding. Only later did we learn that cancer in future offspring can result from this drug: Since 1970 there have been 150 reported cases of vaginal cancer in American girls whose mothers took the drug while pregnant!

Because a few cents' worth implanted in a cow's ear brought more than $12 worth of additional beef, DES continued to be used up to 1973, although animal experiments showed that this chemical caused leukemia, tumors of the testicles, cysts and cancers of the uterus, cervix, and breast, and so on. After more than a decade of widespread use, the FDA, responding to outraged scientific and consumer groups, attempted to ban DES in 1973. But in January, 1974, the U.S. Court of Appeals overturned the ban because there were "disputed facts" about its hazards to health, so today this killer is back in our beef.

Judges, it seems, do not fully comprehend that hormones, as well as vitamins, minerals, hallucinogenic drugs, and other chemical agents can often produce powerful bodily effects, even in the minutest concentrations. Chemical levels barely detectable by the most advanced current laboratory procedures—and perhaps also lesser amounts, undetectable today—may nonetheless deeply affect the human cells, which are a more sensitive biochemical apparatus.

In the case of DES, as in so many other cases, despite strong suspicions from animal experiments of the extreme damage it can cause, we are continuing to use the chemical because our concern for the dollar is stronger than our concern for our health. This is another battle, a continuing battle, in the biochemical civil war we are waging against ourselves—this battle thought to be won in 1973, but now lost again in 1974—and with unknown casualties still to be counted.

Intentional Food Pollution

Some constituents in our food are unintentional, such as residues of fertilizers, pesticides, hormones, tranquilizers, antibiotics, radioactive agents, and other chemicals used in the raising of crops and animals, or part of the damaging wastes of our industrial high-energy society.

Others are used intentionally to treat foods or process them, and should be called *food pollution*. Some examples:

- Boric acid, called "poisonous per se" by the Food and Drug Administration, used to dust hams as a preservative.
- Sodium sulphate, illegally used to restore the color of decaying meat and to remove the strong odor of putrefaction.
- Sodium nitrate and sodium nitrite, which are preservatives and color accentuators for luncheon meats (hot dogs, salamis, bolognas, etc.), smoked fish, bacon, and ham. These are directly toxic to very young children, and excesses can produce severe immediate sicknesses in adults. Perhaps more serious, it has been verified that these may also combine with other chemicals to form the cancer-producing *nitrosamines*. "Cooked bacon invariably contains nitrosamines and is probably the most dangerous food in the supermarket," says microbiologist Michael Jacobson.

Today the hopes of the food industries to continue using nitrates and nitrites (which are especially useful because they retard the development of potentially lethal bacteria in prepared meats) seem to rest on vitamin C, because there is new evidence that this vitamin retards the formation of nitrosamines. A massive study is now under way to verify this protective property. If successful, we can expect to have bacon, smoked ham, hot dogs, etc., soon to be marketed with the slogan VITAMIN C FORTIFIED, with their nitrate or nitrite contents undiminished.

- "U.S. Certified Dyes." This certification is supposed to mean such artificial colors are "pure and unharmful." Formerly there were 19 such certified and widely used dyes, but 8 have since been "decertified," largely because they were proved to be cancer-inducing. Two such dyes, for example, Yellow AB and Yellow OB, were once commonly used to color butter and margarine. They were made from a chemical which, according to a physician formerly with the National Cancer Institute, has "remarkably low toxicity, while being one of the most carcinogenic substances known." This means that although they are not poisonous in the ordinary sense, they are potent cancer-producers.

Another dye still in use is amaranth, called Red No. 2 for short. In 1973 *Medical World News* reported that two years earlier "the Soviet Union banned the coloring on the basis of research implicating it in birth defects, impaired reproduction, and cancer in rats." But in that same year, "the FDA certified for use more than 1.2 million pounds of the dye, which produces the vivid cherry hue of soft drinks and is also added to ice cream, candies, baked goods, and sausages. A popular sugar-coated cornflake is sprayed bright pink with Red No. 2 and promoted to children as an energy-packed breakfast." Red No. 2 is still in wide use.

Another azo dye, Violet No. 1, was banned by the FDA in 1973, when *Medical World News* noted: "Repeatedly

questioned by toxologists in its 22 years of use, the color
was pronounced safe . . . as recently as last November. It
was finally yanked when Japanese studies revealed
strong evidence of carcinogenicity." (As we will later
see, riboflavin, vitamin B2, has been pinpointed as a
main protector against the cancer-producing effects in
animal experiments of azo dyes.)

Such incidents—and they are not uncommon—in which
U.S. standards are below foreign ones have led many
to question the vigilance and dedication with which the
FDA is living up to its legal obligation to protect us
against hazardous foods, additives, and drugs. Its severest
critics maintain the Food and Drug Administration—and
the U.S. Department of Agriculture, with which it shares
responsibility for food and food contaminants—have frequently been less concerned with the health and well-
being of the public than with the profits and well-being of
the large food and drug companies.

Dr. Michael Jacobson, for example, tells us that "many of
the top officials in these agencies are former food industry
executives, and it would be a bit naive to expect them to be
strong critics or strict regulators of industry. The Secretary
of Agriculture, Earl Butz, was vice-president of Ralston
Purina. FDA's Director of the Bureau of Foods formerly
worked for Hunt-Wesson; Libby, McNeill & Libby; and
Ralston Purina. Twenty-two of fifty-two top posts in FDA
are held by men and women who were formerly associated
with regulated industry and other special interest
groups. . . .

"Leaving FDA is another problem. The most lucrative
positions for departing FDA officials are in companies
which the FDA is supposed to regulate. In 1969 a Con-
gressional committee discovered that 37 of 49 recently resigned or retired employees went on to serve regulated industries in various capacities. In August, 1972, the Deputy
Commissioner of FDA quit to become special assistant to

the Chairman of CPC, International, which makes Mazola margarine, Skippy peanut butter, Hellman mayonnaise, among other products ... How is the public to trust its regulatory officials if they are fishing for jobs with the very companies they are supposed to be cracking down on?"

A listing of other intentionally added food pollutants would be too long to give in detail, for it would have to include many other preservatives, and also "stabilizers," imitation flavors (715 in current use), acidifiers, thickeners, emulsifiers, softeners, sweeteners, bleaches, texture enhancers, antifoamers, antisprouting agents, dough conditioners, ripeners, waxes, and so on. Today we each eat about 5 pounds per person per year of 2,500 such additives, which together make up a billion pounds of chemicals poured annually into our foods. Despite the consumer movement and health furor, some have increased greatly in recent years: For example, the average American now eats ten times as much artificial coloring matter than he did in 1940.

Physicians now know with certainty that such additives cause many patients to have allergies, headaches, nasal polyps, asthma, skin lesions, mouth chancres, swellings of the larynx, hyperkinesis, and other behavioral and mental disturbances. Other ill effects, such as cancer, that may arise after years or decades of low-level exposure, are less concretely linked to these often unnecessary food additives, but the evidence of their culpability continues to mount.

Should we then wonder at the declining state of our national health? At our unsatisfactory life expectancy, infant mortality, heart attack, cancer, suicide, stroke, diabetes, high blood pressure, and similar distressing disease rates? Or should we rather wonder why, in case after case, the FDA and the Department of Agriculture have acted too little and too late to protect our health? And could there be a link to the fact, as reported in *The Chemical Feast*, that *"the vitamin content of the American diet is deterio-*

rating"? Later we will see many connections between vitamins and these agents of environmental stress.

The Health Food Movement

The "organic" or "natural" food movement has been rising in popularity as our environment and food supply worsen. The idea is simple: Abandon all chemical agents on the farm (especially pesticides and fertilizers) and use only natural animal manures and composts made from vegetation to condition the soil and feed the plants.

The claim is that these "natural" methods will produce, when properly applied, an abundance of crops. These crops will be healthy and have great nutritive value. Insects and other pests will be less able to attack such "healthy" organically grown plants.

Most knowledgeable and impartial observers who have examined these claims do not agree. They point out that no living things can create minerals, such as iron, copper, iodine, or calcium. A soil deficient in such minerals must have them supplied from an outside source because the manures of animals raised in the locality and composts from local vegetation will also lack the missing minerals. Organic farming methods cannot overcome such a mineral deficiency.

Many experimenters have tested the farm produce that has been grown in various ways for nutritive content, especially vitamin content and the presence of the important protein-building amino acids. It is indisputable that chemical fertilizers can often greatly improve the nutrient content of food crops and add to the health and sturdiness of the plants.

The organic farming proponents are on better grounds as regards chemical pesticides, which are poisons that nobody wishes to use, which do not improve the nutritional quality of any crop, and which are more dangerous to us than most fertilizer residues.

But it is sad to report that many buyers of foods labeled "organically grown" are being hoaxed all over the country. Unscrupulous farmers or merchants are charging higher prices for farm products grown in the ordinary way, pesticides and all, and then mislabeled.

The Connecticut State Consumer Protection Department recently tested 7 foods labeled "organically grown" and found 6 to have residues from pesticide sprays.

In Denver the FDA's tests found such spray residues on many foods labeled and sold as unsprayed at special high prices.

In New York, the state Agriculture Department reported that of 55 products sold as "organic," 30 percent had pesticide residues—as compared with a lower 20 percent among comparable ordinary foods for which no special claim was made!

There are even vitamin supplements being widely sold with an "organic" or "natural" label whose ingredients are largely the ordinary, synthetically produced pure vitamins.

"Rose Hips Vitamin C," for example, is often not what the customer thinks. Rose hips contain only a small amount of vitamin C (approximately 1½ to 2 percent), so these products must be fortified with other vitamin C (usually manufactured by fermentation of corn dextrose) to meet the desired potency.

One vitamin purveyor refuses to use the word "organic." His brochure explains why:

> Because this word is so *misused* today that it *misleads* people. In the early years of the Natural Food movement the words *organically grown* meant (and still mean) that a food was grown on naturally fertilized soil free from harmful sprays or dust. Unfortunately the terminology was shortened to *"Organic"* which permitted another interpretation, namely the chemical one—*a compound containing carbon.* So today we have food products on the market labeled *organic* which means they contain carbon as all

foods do. We have *vitamins* labeled *organic* which simply means they contain *carbon* and all *synthetic vitamins* contain carbon. In fact the following can all correctly be labeled organic: plastics, dacron, detergents, antibiotics, insecticides, etc. Even *Coal Tar* can be legally labeled *natural—organic* because it is a natural substance and it does contain carbon. With this in mind you can understand why we do not use this word on our products. . . .

This is perfectly correct. The technical scientific meaning of the word "organic" does not coincide with the idea most people have, so deception is easy. It is hard to take legal measures against those who sell ordinary foods labeled "organic" at special higher prices to unsuspecting consumers.

But since there are high profits to be made selling vitamins or farm produce this way, it was perhaps inevitable that such deception would appear in the food markets, the health shops, and the vitamin catalogs.

As we shall see, vitamins derived from natural sources are not always superior to those synthesized or manufactured by fermentation; the five to one hundred times higher prices often asked for "all-natural" vitamins are a particularly cruel form of consumer deception, frequently victimizing the elderly, who often most need supplemental vitamins but may be least able to afford unnecessary and wasteful expenditures.

The situation is not so different for food. Truly "natural" foods should mean pure foods—that is, foods free of damaging residues. But it is doubtful or improbable that we can grow enough food in the world for ourselves and other hungry peoples without using toxic pesticides. Insect and other pests are fierce predators. Even with the millions of pounds of chemical poisons now being used in America to protect our food and fiber against them, the best estimate is that we still lose a full 20 percent of our agricultural yields to plant diseases, molds, insects, rodents, and the like. At a special experimental farm in Virginia, even using old-fashioned "pesticides" of the nineteenth century (fermented urine, for example), trial after trial has only produced puny crops or crop failure. Modern pests are just too strong and voracious. The findings of fraud in so-called organically grown foods at special high prices that still have pesticide residues also show the difficulty of raising adequate crops without such poisons.

But the desire for "natural" foods—foods without fertilizer or pesticide *residues*—should not diminish. Perhaps we should begin to call these *pure* foods instead, because the idea of purity, including pure vitamins, pure air and water, comes closer to our bodies' true needs for unadulterated nourishment and healthful environments. Such purity in our total environment could surely bring years and years of additional vigorous life to millions of Americans and prevent large amounts of distressing disease and disability.

But perhaps this is an overly naïve or optimistic hope, even for the future. Nutritional and environmental improvement conflict with our seemingly more-important high-energy, rushed, profit-making "standard of living." Few of us can do much as individuals to alter the habits and practices of our society. But much control of our own bodies is possible.

An ameba, whose single cell is a relative of human cells, responds to need automatically, its nutrition and maturation being governed exactly by its immediate environment and its inherent biochemical coding. The cells of a human being are encased in a body and depend solely on the intake of that body for sustenance. Office patients are frequently told: "Feed your cells and sustain yourself." Every requirement of the human body, operating on a twenty-four-hour cycle, must so be met. It is a rare individual who can do this adequately in our age of nonnutritious foodstuffs and a waste-contaminated environment. The supplementation of vitamins can be a major aid against the havoc that has been created with our physical and mental status.

With all this evidence of the nutritional degradation of our food supply and the contamination of our resources of air, water, and land, it becomes more and more obvious how important vitamins and other nutritional supplements are to our personal health.

CHAPTER 7:

The Unfinished Medical
History of Vitamins

Though vitamins are very much on the frontiers of current biomedical science, they also go back thousands of years in human history. Among the earliest medical records that survive are those of a dreaded and often formerly fatal malady feared for over two millennia—scurvy.

Scurvy

Long ago Hippocrates himself, the ancient father of medicine, mentioned the debility, bleeding gums, and hemorrhages of scurvy, found in cities under siege and armies existing for long periods on dried rations. It was later reported that during the Crusades the defeat and capture of St. Louis and all his knights was due to scurvy.

As the age of great ocean explorations by slow sailing ships began, this disease was to ravage the early Portuguese and Spanish explorers who had no fresh food. One hundred of a total crew of 160 perished of scurvy during the famous voyage of Vasco da Gama in 1497–98, and in 1577 a Spanish galleon was found adrift with all aboard dead of this malady.

It is also told that a group of Portuguese sailors on one of Columbus' voyages were in the final stages of scurvy and asked to be put ashore to die on land. They were left on a passing island, where hunger drove them to eat wild plants and fruits. Later their vessel returned by the same route, and their shipmates were astonished to find them recovered and in good health. The island later came to be called Curaçao, meaning "cure" in Portuguese, and eventually became the source of the sweet liqueur of that name, made from oranges.

Sailing men continued to succumb in great numbers to scurvy—more died of this disease, according to one writer, than in all the naval battles of history—until about a century ago, even though the Scotch physician James Lind published his important *Treatise on Scurvy* in 1753. In it he described his experiments showing how scurvy could be overcome by citrus fruits, but a half century passed until the British Navy in 1795 ordered a daily ration of citrus juice for its seamen (giving rise to the "Limey" nickname they have carried ever since). Many years later, similar measures were taken for merchant seamen, and finally the dreaded scurvy began to disappear from the history of maritime affairs.

Scurvy begins gradually, with a general debility, or weakness, and restlessness. Then sunken eyes, a sallow complexion, tender gums, and muscular pains follow. In 80 percent of the cases there is anemia. Owing to weakness in the capillaries (the smallest blood vessels), the gums begin to bleed and there is a tendency to bruise easily. This may continue, gradually worsening for weeks or months as hemorrhages appear in the tissues, the bones weaken, the teeth fall out, and the gums protrude. Night blindness and other visual disorders may also occur. The bones may become so brittle that they break with normal movements. Finally, a deep exhaustion overtakes the sufferer and complications, such as lung and kidney troubles, lead to death.

Long before death, however, the general weaknesses of scurvy can be seriously incapacitating. Before the work of Lind was put into effect in the British Royal Navy, for example, seagoing combat fleets had to be relieved every ten weeks to replace the weakened seamen with a fresh crew. In his important 1972 book, *The Healing Factor: Vitamin C Against Disease*, the biochemist and modern vitamin C pioneer Irwin Stone points out that the work of Lind was as important in breaking the power of Napoleon as Admiral Nelson himself. With their seamen fortified against scurvy, "the English vessels were able to maintain continuous blockade duties, laying off the coast of France for months at a time without the necessity of relieving the men. Were it not for Lind, the flat-bottomed invasion barges assembled by Napoleon may well have crossed the English channel."

Today we know that scurvy is caused purely and simply by a lack of vitamin C (ascorbic acid) and can be cured at almost all stages by the administration of the vitamin, by injection or orally in chemical form, or as a constituent of fresh fruits and vegetables.

Vitamin C dissolves readily in water, and excess amounts that are eaten are easily excreted in the urine. The body does not store large amounts of this vitamin, yet severe signs of a deficiency do not appear immediately when vitamin C is missing from the diet. Subtle signs of borderline deficiency begin to appear slowly, such as "pink toothbrush" and visible minor bruises. Growing teeth in children are affected, and bones may lose elasticity and strength.

Except for extreme and exceptional conditions, such as those experienced by the American prisoners-of-war in North Vietnam (many of whom did contract the early stages of scurvy), this disease is a rarity in modern life. But minor vitamin C insufficiences do occur, especially among the elderly, whose poor teeth may inhibit the eating of fruit or whose diets may be poor owing to low income or loneliness.

Scurvy was only one of dozens and dozens of mysterious afflictions to our ancestors. Great plagues and epidemics, lingering and wasting fevers, and inexplicable deformities in growing children were all commonplace. Those were the days when a majority of all children did not reach adolescence: As late as 1800 nearly half of all newborn infants failed to reach their tenth year. We sometimes tend to overlook the great progress medicine has made since those times.

Though it was known how to prevent or alleviate scurvy in the nineteenth century, nothing was then understood about the cause of the disease—or, indeed, of most other human afflictions. This understanding was only to come much later, as a result of investigations of another deficiency disease.

Beriberi and the Discovery of Deficiency Diseases

Beriberi, once also called polyneuritis, began to be noticed in the Western world long after scurvy because it was widespread only in the rice-eating areas of the world. Where polished rice became the staple food—in India, South China, the Philippine Islands, the Dutch East Indies, and parts of South America and Japan—this severe and fatal malady appeared.

Beriberi is the Ceylonese word for weakness, and its other symptoms include gastric irritation, extreme emaciation, a swelling of the legs, chest, and face, and a painful degeneration of the nerves. Congestive heart failure or a paralytic inability to breathe can then cause death.

At the time when beriberi came to Western attention, medical science was already in the flush of extraordinary change. Pasteur had promulgated the "germ theory" in 1877, a startling and profound event in the history of medicine. This came only after several centuries of slow discovery: The compound microscope had been invented three hundred years earlier in Holland by Janssen in 1590, but it was ninety-three years after that before his countryman Anton van Leeuwenhoek produced the first pictorial representation of bacteria—and then another century passed until Edward Jenner in 1796 in England discovered that man could be protected against disfiguring and often fatal smallpox by inoculation with cowpox (a weaker form of the disease), similar to a remedy that was already being applied in the Turkish world.

In Europe, in the first part of the nineteenth century, great strides were being made in surgery by dedicated scientists, including the use of anesthesia and a recognition of the importance of antisepsis (a clean or sterile environment) for successful operations. Often these medical pioneers faced skepticism and ridicule at first. Such was also the first response to Pasteur's germ theory of 1877, stating that microorganisms could cause human disease.

Pasteur, a chemist rather than a physician, had been led to his conclusions by studies of fermentation and anthrax, and he was later to apply them dramatically to rabies. He and the other great medical pioneers of the time—Joseph Lister, Robert Koch, Emil von Behring, and others—truly revolutionized medical thinking. Mysterious scourges such as cholera, diphtheria, typhoid, tuberculosis, and other infectious maladies that had plagued mankind for centuries could now be comprehended for the first time.

After the initial skepticism that greets any new idea was overcome, extensive searches began to find the microbes responsible for various diseases, to study these germs and their action within and outside the body, and to generate countermeasures against them, especially protective vaccines. (A vaccine, such as those now widely used against smallpox, polio, measles, etc., stimulates the body to produce protective substances, called antibodies, that can later overcome invading microorganisms or viruses.) Many successes were achieved, but it was not to be until much later, until the 1940's, that antibiotics (chemical agents that themselves directly attack hostile microbes in the body) came to be applied against infectious diseases.

Thus it is not surprising that the first investigators of beriberi in the late nineteenth century concentrated their efforts on finding a microbe responsible for the disorder.

Such were the specific instructions given to the young Dutch physician Christian Eijkman sent to the East Indies in 1886 to investigate the disease. After several years of little progress, he noticed, in a fortuitous accident now famous in the history of nutritional research, that a mysterious occurrence had taken place among the chickens in the laboratory compound.

For a time the chickens had also been stricken with a strange fatal paralysis similar to beriberi, which then just as suddenly ceased to affect them. An inquiry showed that some months earlier, the chickens had been placed on a diet of polished rice, the more expensive grains from which the outer husk is removed. This took place before the onset of the malady. Then a new cook, wishing to economize, switched back to the cheaper, unpolished rice, whereupon the disease promptly disappeared.

The concept of a deficiency disease did not exist at the time, though several, notably Dr. Charles Hose, were suggesting that beriberi was related to diet. Many thought something in the food offered protection against a germ, and this protection was removed when the rice was refined. Another theory was that it was not a germ but a poison that produced the disease—a poison in the polished rice that was normally counteracted by a naturally occurring antidote in the husk. Take away the husk and the poison (or a germ) would take over and cause beriberi.

Gradually, by 1907, a much simpler concept evolved, that there was an essential *nutrient* in the discarded rice polishings whose absence caused beriberi. Research was later to discover that this was the vitamin thiamin (vitamin B_1), so minutely present that a ton (2,000 lbs.) of unpolished rice contains only a fraction of a pound of thiamin.

During this time, roughly from 1880 to 1910, biochemists in several nations were demonstrating that mice and rats fed a diet of pure protein, carbohydrates, fats, and minerals would succumb to disability or disease. Some additional natural food, such as milk or eggs, was necessary for their proper growth, reproduction, and health. Scurvy could not be induced in mice and rats because, as was discovered later, they can manufacture vitamin C themselves. But in 1907 researchers did produce scurvy in the guinea pig, the only small laboratory animal that requires vitamin C in its diet.

Then, in 1911, after the British investigators Henry Fraser and Ambrose Stanton had also proposed that beriberi was caused by a dietary deficiency, the Polish biochemist Casimir Funk working in London isolated from rice polishings a beriberi-preventive agent. He coined the word "vitamine," and the vitamin theory was born.

As we said before, the idea of the vitamin theory is that minute amounts of certain organic chemical compounds are necessary in the diet for health. This became firmly established in medicine only when experiments with animals were devised that showed conclusively that dietary deficiencies could cause disease.

Other Vitamins Discovered and the Cause of Rickets

Many such experiments were then begun, as investigators rushed to apply the new theory. In short order, vitamin A, other B vitamins, and the anti-scurvy vitamin (called vitamin C before its chemical nature was known) began to be recognized.

Rickets was a troubling bone deformity among infants that had also been known since antiquity. Grotesquely bowed and weakened legs, deformities of the skull and chest shape, and other skeletal signs appear in babies with rickets. Those who had puzzled over the condition had noted that it never appeared among "primitive" peoples but seemed to be a by-product of civilization.

In 1919 an investigator produced the disorder in dogs and then showed that it could be cured or prevented by cod-liver oil, thus demonstrating that it was, in fact, a deficiency disease. But he believed that the newly discovered vitamin A was the active agent. Three years later, other researchers showed that the protective power of cod-liver oil against rickets survived heating and aeration of the oil (which destroy vitamin A), so it was clear that a new substance was involved, and this was named vitamin D. Later it would be learned that except for certain fish-liver oils, vitamin D is hardly to be found in any other naturally occurring foodstuff but is created on the human skin by the action of sunlight, which is apparently how nature intended the human infant to receive it.

As time passed, additional vitamins were discovered, and their biochemical and biological properties probed more deeply. The honor roll of scientists who spent their working lifetimes on this important research includes many dedicated workers from different countries, several later to be awarded Nobel Prizes and other awards. Such researchers as E. V. McCollum, M. Davis, T. B. Osborne, L. B. Mendel, Paul Gyorgy, H. M. Evans, K. S. Bishop, H. Dam, T. Mellanby, A. Szent-Györgyi, P. Karrer, Roger J. Williams, and many others contributed greatly to this important field.

After the first recognition of the existence of a vitamin, the procedure is for investigators to attempt to isolate it in pure form and then to identify its chemical composition. Following that, chemists try to synthesize or manufacture it in the laboratory. These steps can take many, many years and extraordinary labor.

For example, it was not until 1933, twenty years after its first recognition, that the chemical nature of vitamin A was firmly established, and then it took until 1947 until it could be synthesized. Vitamin B_{12}, whose lack causes pernicious anemia, a chronic and progressive anemia of older adults and vegetarians, was isolated in 1948, but its synthesis took the efforts of 99 workers from 19 countries over an 11-year period, in a major project jointly directed from Harvard and Zurich.

Vitamin Research

Discovery, isolation, and synthesis are only part of vitamin research. Most important is learning how vitamins work in human and animal bodies.

To do this, one fundamental approach is to deprive animals—and, with proper safeguards, also human volunteers—of a vitamin and examine the effects. Also parts of the body can be examined for vitamin content. And radioactive tracers are added to "tag" vitamins when they are fed, so their progress in the body can be followed and their functions understood.

Then vitamins are administered in varying doses. This can be under normal conditions or with known preexisting disease or injury. Or, disease-causing agents can be given simultaneously, to see whether the vitamins have any protective effect. From such work the cancer-retarding properties of vitamins have been learned, as well as their preventive powers against cardiovascular and other diseases.

Many questions, even of a basic nature, remain to be answered. Some have to do with the existence of vitamins. It is not fully agreed upon that certain substances—PABA, inositol, the bioflavonoids (vitamin P), pangamic acid (vitamin B_{16}), vitamin B_{14}, and the new vitamin Q—are truly vitamins. There remain wide differences of opinion. (Russian scientists, by the way, accord vitamin status to more of these controversial substances than most American physicians and also recommend and use vitamins therapeutically to a greater extent. Life expectancy in the Soviet Union ranks just behind our own—and they are catching up fast.) And, of course, other vitamins may still be undiscovered because they are only needed in ultraminute quantities.

One factor complicating the situation is that the body can often meet its needs for a particular vitamin by using slightly different substances. Usually these are closely related molecules, chemical cousins, so to speak. For example, the protein amino acid tryptophan can be converted, in certain amounts, into niacin (vitamin B3) by the body. Also, both *nicotinic acid* and *nicotinamide* (also called *niacinamide*) work as vitamin B3, and both of these are called niacin. Similarly, Vitamin B6 activity can come from any one of three substances (pyridoxine, pyridoxal, or pyridoxamine), all of which are closely related.

The Minute Quantities

Another complicating factor is the very small quantities involved. Most of the vitamins that dissolve readily in water—the "water-soluble" group, consisting of vitamin C and all the B vitamins—are measured in *milligrams*. One milligram is 1/1,000 of a gram. A gram itself is a small unit of weight, about 1/28 of an ounce. (This is the weight of about one-quarter teaspoon of vitamin C crystals.)

When the pure substance becomes available, working with the tiny quantities necessary is less difficult than one would think. For example, take a quarter teaspoon of vitamin C crystals, about 1 gram, and dissolve this in a quart of pure water. There are about 200 teaspoons in a quart, so each teaspoon of the solution just created has about 1/200 of a gram, or 5/1,000 of a gram, or 5 milligrams of vitamin C. This is usually abbreviated "5 mg."

Let's go one step further. Take a teaspoon of this first solution and add it to a second quart of pure water and mix thoroughly. Now each teaspoon of the second quart has 5/200 or 25/1,000 of a milligram of the original vitamin. A little work with fractions will show you this is the same as 25/1,000,000, or 25 millionths of a gram. These units, millionths of a gram, are called *micrograms* and abbreviated "mcg" or "μmg." Micrograms are the units used to measure vitamin B12.

There are four fat-soluble vitamins. These are vitamins A, D, E, and K. They dissolve in oils and fats, rather than water, and can be stored up in the body, unlike the water-soluble B vitamins and vitamin C, of which only small bodily reserves can exist. The fat-soluble vitamins are not measured in units of weight, such as milligrams and micrograms. Instead, *International Units* (IU's) are used for these vitamins. The amount (by weight) of vitamin in one IU varies from vitamin to vitamin. Vitamins A and D are very potent, and one IU for each of these contains only micrograms of the chemical substance that is the vitamin. Vitamin E is needed in larger amounts, and in this case one IU is actually the same as one mg.

Minerals and Other Nutrients

Nutritional research has also discovered other nutrients whose lack in our diet can cause health problems. Many minerals are of course also essential, and these must be eaten for good health. Calcium, phosphorus, sodium, and potassium are needed in relatively large amounts, measured in grams. Iron, magnesium, copper, and zinc are needed in milligram amounts and iodine in microgram quantities. It is known that the body also requires chlorine, sulfur, fluorine, and manganese in small trace quantities, and there is evidence to indicate a need for chromium, cobalt, selenium, and molybdenum as well.

Protein is the building block of the body. Ingested proteins are broken down into simpler components called amino acids. Twenty of these amino acids are known to be in the human body. In re-forming protein from food to build our body cells, hair, nails, and so on, it turns out that only 8 amino acids must be in the adult diet (infants need more). These amino acids are thus also essential nutrients for good health.

Similarly, the brain cannot function well without a small supply of the natural sugar glucose, which the body most readily furnishes from carbohydrates (fruit sugars or starches) in the diet.

And there are also certain fats, called Essential Fatty

Acids (EFA) that are required for proper functioning. (Some writers have called these vitamin F because they are also only needed in small quantities, but this name is not widely used.)

It should not be surprising that such a bewildering variety of food nutrients are needed, because nutrition is such a basic part of the extraordinarily complex phenomenon we call life.

Nor, reviewing this thumbnail history of vitamins, should it be surprising that it is an unfinished history, with great discoveries now being made and others that lie ahead. We are at the threshold of our understanding, especially about the ways in which vitamins function inside the body and about the effects of various vitamin intakes. These are often the subject of much controversy—a beneficial controversy, for without it little progress would be made.

As in many fields of human activity, it often takes time, sometimes years or decades, for new advances in medicine to be understood and properly applied. Penicillin, for example, was first discovered in 1929, but it was not until the 1940's and the stimulus of World War II that it began to be used as an antibiotic against many infectious diseases. The new vitamin knowledge, the result of research that has spurted ahead in just the past few years, offers similar great promise for human betterment as this knowledge is verified and applied.

The history of vitamins continues, and, throughout, the evidence grows that the role of vitamins in human health has changed significantly. In earlier times, this role was to overcome disorders owing to outright deficiencies. Now we look more toward the role that vitamins can play in preventive medicine, by aiding the body and mind to withstand outside assaults, and by boosting the chances for robust health.

8:

Vitamin Deficiencies and High-Level Therapeutic Dosages

Low-level vitamin supplements have been taken by many millions of people for decades, usually to little effect. The most widely sold supplements, even the so-called therapeutic types, provide small amounts of vitamins, perhaps up to two or three times the recommended daily minimal allowances. But there is mounting evidence that many conditions exist for which higher vitamin dosages of tenfold to hundredfold amounts are not only effective but necessary.

Anemic Monkeys

To help understand why such high dosages are often essential, let us consider an illustrative experiment performed by Dr. Coy D. Fitch, now of the Department of Internal Medicine and Biochemistry in St. Louis, and reported in the 1968 issue of *Vitamins and Hormones*. He and his colleagues, working earlier at the University of Arkansas, used the rhesus monkey, an experimental animal closer to man than other animals, such as rats and mice, that are more often used in nutrition research.

In this experiment, 32 young monkeys were fed a vitamin E-deficient diet for a long period, while 30 similar monkeys received the same diet supplemented with vitamin E.

Dr. Fitch wrote:

> On routine examination, Vitamin E-deficient monkeys
> *appear normal for 5–30 months.* Although they do not
> reach puberty, they may at first even match the growth
> rate of their Vitamin E-supplemented counterparts. Even-
> tually, though, there is an abrupt onset of rapidly progres-
> sive weight loss . . . and anemia . . . *Within one to two
> months of this abrupt change, untreated monkeys die.*
> The same devastating disease occurs in response to each
> of the Vitamin E-deficient diets, and it runs the same
> course regardless of whether the onset is at 5 or 30 months
> . . . Vitamin E may be practically undetectable in blood
> serum for two years before the onset of the disease.
> [Emphasis added.]

There was no evidence of heart, kidney, or lung disease,
or any sign of muscle pain or neurological disorder, but the
affected monkeys became too weak to stand without support. Every vitamin E-deficient monkey succumbed so
abruptly to anemia, despite the fact that in some cases,
there were no clinical signs of the deficiency for up to two
and a half years.

This experiment vividly shows the life-and-death importance of vitamin E in an animal close to man and also
demonstrates *that severe vitamin deficiencies can arise
without overt or evident signs.*

That vitamin deficiencies can develop so slowly and un-
noticeably is not a new discovery. In its 1953 edition, the
Encyclopaedia Britannica noted:

> Deficiency diseases are slow to develop because time is
> required to deplete bodily stores of the vitamins. Adult
> animals may ingest a deficient diet for a number of months
> or even years before signs of the disease appear. The time
> required for the development of the disorder varies for
> different vitamins. Manifestastions of a lack of thiamin
> [vitamin B1] develop relatively soon, whereas those of to-

copherol [vitamin E] or Vitamin A deprivation may require a major fraction of the lifespan to become noticeable.

Further, in experiments beginning in the late 1940's, Dr. L. Greenberg and Dr. J. F. Rinehart in San Francisco produced arteriosclerosis in monkeys by a vitamin B6 (pyridoxine) deficient diet. The monkeys got lesions in their arteries after being on the diet from 5½ to 16 months. The doctors wrote: "The experimental lesions . . . have a close resemblance to arteriosclerosis as it occurs in man. . . . It is noteworthy that *pyridoxine deficiency is in essence a chronic deficiency, relatively slow in evolution and without distinctive external manifestations. Such a deficiency state would be one particularly difficult of clinical recognition."* [Emphasis added.]

This research was repeated and verified by other investigators at the Merck Company laboratories and also at the Nagoya University School of Medicine in Japan.

Here may lie part of an explanation to the puzzle of the efficacy of vitamin therapy, especially for persons without clinically evident deficiency diseases—those whose complaints of depression or lack of vitality or anxiety have usually been ascribed to neurosis, hypochondria, or unknown psychosomatic factors. Can it be that many such persons with no overt signs of disease actually have subclinical vitamin deficiencies of long standing? If so, then normal "minimal" vitamin doses might be insufficient to overcome these deficiencies, just as they are insufficient for the standard medical therapeutic treatment of recognized vitamin deficiency diseases.

Morning Sickness and Nausea

We can glean additional theoretical insight into the deficiency problem by noting that there do appear, from time to time, clinically evident cases of actual vitamin deficiencies in our society. These include scurvy (lack of vitamin C), pellagra (niacin, vitamin B₃), and night blindness (vitamin A). Hospitals in large cities do report such cases occasionally, and they are not only among the poor. They also occur among students who eat unwisely, alcoholics, food faddists on exotic diets, those who undertake foolish crash weight-loss programs, and older or single persons who live alone and do not take the trouble to prepare nourishing meals.

At times the effects can be severe, including heart palpitations, chest and abdominal pains, edema (swelling) in the lower limbs, breathlessness, nausea, total exhaustion, and so on. These can often result in hospital admission.

From the existence of such cases—half a dozen or more reported by one large public big city hospital each year —we can deduce that lesser degrees of vitamin insufficiency must also exist because the hospitalized cases are just the tip of the iceberg. Some unknown part of the population *must* be walking about in milder deficiency states, and still more *must* have low vitamin reserves. These lesser insufficiencies can produce less evident symptoms —perhaps downcast feelings, minor bodily weaknesses, an inability to think clearly, a proneness to infections and diseases, and so on. Such effects of malnourishment can readily be found in all sectors of American society.

For example morning sickness is a very common minor affliction in our society. Yet it seems unlikely that the human organism evolved over millions of years so that morning sickness should be a normal, or "natural," part of life. Now there is new clinical evidence that pyridoxine (vitamin B₆) in doses approximately ten to twenty times higher than the recommended minimal daily allowance of 2.5 mg. can often prevent this nausea of pregnancy.

And once morning sickness has begun, still higher doses, one hundred or more times higher than the recommended allowance, can often alleviate it. (This vitamin, as all the other water-soluble B vitamins, is virtually harmless in any dosage.)

In nature, the B vitamins are often found together as a complex of vitamins in such foods as the whole wheat grain, in liver and yeast, and so on.

If primitive woman did not experience morning sickness by virtue of her diet, and vitamin B$_6$ is an "index" of the needed amount of the whole B complex, then this is additional evidence that our vitamin standards are far too low. Eating a natural diet sufficiently high to raise the vitamin B$_6$ level above the point where morning sickness is produced would also have tended to supply the other B vitamins in amounts much greater than we eat or that are officially recommended today.

We also now know that high-level vitamin regimens are frequently helpful in other situations. Nausea is a physiological reaction to emotion, foreign elements, or internal trauma. Pyridoxine (B$_6$) has often also been found to be beneficial for postoperative nausea, nausea arising from radiation therapy, and nausea after exposure to military gases. (Dr. John M. Ellis, a physician in practice in Texas, describes many other promising directions for pyridoxine therapy—for rheumatism, edema (swellings), kidney stones, heart cases, and so on—in his 1973 book, *Vitamin B$_6$: The Doctor's Report*, written with James Presley.)

We noted above that morning sickness can often be prevented by a daily regimen of 50 milligrams (mg) or more of pyridoxine. Once morning sickness has begun, a corrective or restorative dosage of 300 mg can be helpful. In fact, Dr. Ellis, in his practice, recommends a minimal 50 mg for all adults except pregnant women, who should have at least 100 to 300 mg, he feels. It is now also known that about half of the women suffering deleterious effects, especially depression, from birth control pills can be benefited by high intakes of pyridoxine.

Note the difference between these amounts: the 2.5 mg recommended minimal allowance and the 300 mg restorative or therapeutic dosage. Such hundredfold variation is not uncommon in dealing with the water-soluble vitamins. Providing such large intakes is believed to "saturate the tissues" throughout the body, which is important because these vitamins are known to be needed by every living cell, and the high dosages are medically harmless to those in normal health.

Thus we can list several separate strands of evidence that point to a hitherto unsuspected need for high-level vitamin supplements. We know that vitamin deficiencies causing actual physical damage may be long-term and virtually unrecognizable. We also know that certain widespread minor complaints like morning sickness can be overcome by high-level vitamin doses; this leads us to the conclusion that our vitamin standards may be too low. We suspect that deficiency states may also be widespread. And we know that the professional treatment of a recognized vitamin deficiency (in a hospital or physician's office) does involve high-level vitamin therapy, with dosages far above the minimal recommendations.

Pellagra: the Deficiency Killer

There should have been more of a clue to the general value of high-level vitamin regimens some fifty years ago when researchers first discovered that pellagra was caused by a vitamin deficiency.

Pellagra is a distressing and mortal ailment, first noted in Italy and Spain, and at one time common in the southern section of the United States when a large part of the diet consisted of corn or corn products. This food lacks the needed vitamin *niacin* (B3) and is also low in a certain amino acid that the body can partly convert to niacin.

Sufferers from pellagra may have headaches, diarrhea, giddiness, singing in the ears, and, often, a rash with painful red spots. Mental disorders appear early, and they continue and worsen. In later stages the skin shrivels, the muscles waste, and the patient succumbs—if untreated.

Medical school jargon called it the disease of the 4 D's—Dermatitis, Diarrhea, Dementia, and Death. Included among the signs of the "dementia" may be nervousness, insomnia, loss of memory, irritability, confusion, depression, hallucinations, and so on.

In 1925 Dr. Joseph Goldberger of the U.S. Public Health Service, after a decade of heroic work, proved that pellagra is caused by a nutritional deficiency, and later Dr. Tom Spies and others pioneered in its treatment, using brewers' yeast, a rich source of niacin and other B vitamins, to supplement a nutritious diet. (There is little niacin in cow's milk, by the way, so infants have often suffered from this deficiency, the first major observable sign being diarrhea.)

The interesting clue is that while the normal amount of this vitamin supposedly needed by each of us every day is only 5 mg to 20 mg (thousandths of a gram), depending on age and weight, it was found that massive daily doses of 600 or more milligrams often are required to cure pellagra. This is many times the tiny amount of the recommended daily requirement. Further, long after their symptoms are relieved, former pellagra patients may continue to need such large vitamin doses; otherwise their symptoms may recur.

Thus to bring a vitamin-deficient sick person back to health, extra-large vitamin doses may be required, *and these doses may have to be continued long after overt signs of the deficiency are gone.* Evidently, by some as yet not completely understood mechanism, a deficiency state can induce higher than normal future needs for vitamins.

Scurvy and Vitamin C

We can understand more about the need for higher-than-minimal vitamin quantities for restorative purposes from some findings about scurvy reported in the *Journal of the American Geriatric Society* in 1970. In a hospital geriatric ward, examinations had disclosed that many of the elderly had hitherto undetected signs of mild scurvy. Anemia, painful limbs, and many bruises not caused by bumps or falls were among the signs and symptoms.

A daily dosage of 700 mg of vitamin C was begun. The daily minimal intake of vitamin C required to prevent a clinically recognizable deficiency is generally believed to be only 10 mg, so these patients were being administered seventy times the preventive amount.

Their urine was examined regularly for vitamin C. Despite the high dosage, it took *three weeks* for the vitamin to appear in the urine, indicating that all the vitamin given earlier had been absorbed or used. Presumably, during this three-week period, the body's reserves of vitamin C were being restored, and the bodily tissues saturated with it. A relatively large amount of vitamin C for several weeks was thus needed to overcome the deficiency.

Cellular Malnutrition

Pellagra and scurvy are serious deficiency diseases, while morning sickness is a minor and transitory complaint. But in all of these cases the disorder could have been prevented by a certain vitamin intake. Furthermore, once the disorder was established, a much larger quantity of the vitamin was necessary for treatment.

A similar relationship appears to apply to the vitamin needs of persons without definite signs of any deficiency, but who may have inadequate or marginal vitamin intakes at present or who may have had such poor nutrition in the past. High-level doses seem to be needed for full restorative effect.

Even when there is no observable damage or clinical sign, vitamin reserves may still be low owing to long periods of inadequate intake. This is known from many animal experiments and also from autopsies on human beings in which bodily organs are examined for vitamin content. Studies show, for example, that accident victims have higher vitamin A reserves in the liver (where more than 90 percent of the body's vitamin A is stored) than persons who succumb to infectious diseases. Since those who have accidental deaths can be presumed to be in normal health on the average (or closer to it than the diseased), this links vitamin A depletion closely to such infectious diseases.

Vitamin A is known to be important for the well-being of the epithelial membranes, which are the tissues that line the respiratory tract and whose mucus flow can flush away hostile microorganisms. Many of these cells have tiny hairs, called cilia, which beat in motion, also to move foreign particles away. When these tissues are well nourished and function properly, it is not surprising that there is less infection and greater general health.

A recent major study involved autopsies in five Canadian cities. A total of 500 cadavers, representing a wide span of ages of people who had been in various conditions of health, were examined for vitamin A content. To the surprise of the investigators, nearly one-third of the bodies examined had deficient vitamin A reserves—in Montreal some 20 percent of the autopsied people had no detectable vitamin A reserves in their livers at all.

Since it was believed that most Canadians and Americans had been receiving an adequate vitamin A intake in their food, the researchers suggested that insecticides such as DDT might be responsible for the low or nonexistent vitamin A levels in the livers of so many persons. Such pollutants are believed also to be stored in the liver, where vitamin A combats their harmful presence and is used up in the process.

What could be the general health result of insufficient vitamin intake or inadequate reserves? In many cases there may be no clinical manifestation of deficiency, but today we know that damaging cellular malnutrition may still be occurring. "One can appear perfectly normal in looks and behavior and yet be the victim of mild cellular malnutrition, which may impair the activity of important functioning tissues and decrease one's bodily efficiency materially," writes Professor Roger J. Williams, the discoverer of pantothenic acid, former president of the American Chemical Society, and trustee of the International Academy of Preventive Medicine.

The human body is made up of billions and billions of cells of many types. Every one of these living cells requires an unending supply of nourishment. Every one of them must have vitamins and minerals to live. When these cells are malnourished, so is the body (and mind). "Cellular malnutrition is the basis for all malnutrition," notes Dr. Neil Solomon. In response to the question: *What is the single most important thing I can do for my body?"* his answer, based on a decade of research, is: "To prevent this damaging cellular malnutrition, a well-balanced diet is most important, and this is why you must pay close attention to the food you eat."

Vitamins are indeed foods and a truly well-balanced diet today must include supplements for the proper nourishment of nearly all people. If we neglect our cellular health by allowing deficiencies to build up, the results can be drastic as we shall see in the next chapter, which describes "acquired vitamin dependency."

CHAPTER 9:

Acquired Vitamin Dependency: The Hong Kong Veterans and the Great Depression

In cases where an individual does need a higher-than-average intake of one or more vitamins to be in good health, such a condition may have been present at birth (which we will discuss in the next chapter) or it may be an "acquired vitamin dependency." Here "acquired" means that some peculiarity in past life circumstances, especially a case of malnutrition, has resulted in the body (and mind) having such special vitamin needs.

This concept of acquired vitamin dependency has been advanced by several physicians and investigators, including Yale's Dr. Leon E. Rosenberg, Dr. Abram Hoffer, and this author. At a 1972 Conference on Aging, Dr. Hoffer (as reported in Ruth Adams' and Frank Murray's informative book, *Body, Mind, and the B Vitamins*) described the idea.

"This means that a particular patient requires larger quantities of a particular vitamin than the average person, so that he might require up to one thousand times more than what is average, normal, and optimal for another person. . . . Now, when humans are deprived over a period of many years of the proper nutritional supplements, especially of vitamins, in time they are converting themselves into an acquired dependency condition." In commenting on aging in particular, he added: "I think that what senility is, in fact, is merely a prolonged form of malnutrition."

99

He illustrated the concept by describing the "Hong Kong veterans." These were the survivors of a group of 2,000 Canadian Army men captured at Hong Kong by the Japanese in World War II, and who then endured forty-four months in a rigorous and harsh prisoner-of-war camp. "Most of the men who survived—and there was a fantastically high death rate—came out having lost one-third of their weight and they had in the meantime suffered pellagra, beriberi, many infections and just about every deficiency disease known."

When the war ended in 1945 and they were released, the survivors were hospitalized and treated with what were at the time believed to be large corrective vitamin doses, such as a daily supplement of 50 mg of niacin, about two and a half times the recommended daily allowance. But for many, disturbing symptoms continued for years or decades, and these veterans have been a constant trial to the Canadian government.

Their continuing symptoms included apathy, a cold intolerance of others, fatigue, anxiety, depression, irritability, peptic ulcer, arteriosclerosis, a 70 percent higher coronary death rate than a comparable group who had not suffered such imprisonment, and so on.

Later, one of the Hong Kong veterans who had been afflicted with depression, arthritis, neuritis, and fatigue, became a friend of Dr. Hoffer. In 1960, fifteen years after the war had ended, Dr. Hoffer began to treat the veteran without knowing his full background, as part of a research project at the geriatric clinic. The treatment began with 3 gm (3,000 mg) of niacin daily, which is about two hundred times the recommended dietary allowance. Two weeks later the man had become normal.

But he continued to need the high daily niacin intake. Once in the following twelve years, up to 1972, the patient left his vitamins behind on a long absence and found his disturbing symptoms recurring. When he returned home and went back to the vitamin regimen, they disappeared again.

In all, twelve of the survivors of the Hong Kong veterans have now had similar vitamin therapy, and all of these are now normal, according to Dr. Hoffer.

One cannot help being reminded of the more recent return from North Vietnamese prison camps of the American POW's in 1973 and of the reported cases of depression, alienation, and suicide among some of these men.

During their captivity, many of these prisoners were aware of the dangers of extreme malnutrition, and they knew that scurvy, beriberi, and other deficiency signs (night blindness, edema, diarrhea) were occurring among them.

After they were released, one prisoner reported: "Since our capitivity diet varied from adequate to a starvation level, we were always eager to find some way to improve our vitamin intake. All of the American prisoners were aware of the dangers of scurvy. Sometimes we could gather wild elderberries. Also, we'd try eating leaves, especially those that tasted sour."

Very few of us have had to face such rigors. Our bodies have not been subjected to the challenges of extreme starvation-level malnutrition. In fact, most of us have never been hungry or malnourished at all—or have we?

The Great Depression

In 1935 I. G. Schlink wrote of the immediately past years of great economic depression: "Only about 10 percent of the population received an income which permits them to eat good, well-selected foods in adequate amounts." The medical writer Paul de Kruif lamented in 1936 that "malnourished wretchedness among children is widespread, notorious . . ."; and the Children's Bureau, investigating in Atlanta, Memphis, Racine, Terre Haute, and elsewhere, found that one-fifth of the families were subsisting almost exclusively "on bread, beans, and potatoes."

A few years earlier, Congressman Huddleston had claimed that "men are actually starving by the thousands today, children are being stunted by lack of food. . . ."

In our vitamin and nutritional controversies today, we may have limited our vision unnecessarily to just the current conditions. The cases of clinical pellagra patients, the Hong Kong veterans, and the American POW's show that past nutritional circumstances in an individual's life may have an important bearing on his or her present vitamin needs.

We especially overlook the fact that all Americans who are now over 35 years of age did live through some or all of the Great Depression. Those who are now 35 to 60 spent part of their formative and growing years, between birth and age 16, during that unhappy era when many ate so poorly. The consequences of such a time of mass national malnutrition have never been adequately measured, for the society or for an individual. For many adults, in fact, the circumstances of that time may be lost to memory, buried in the "childhood amnesia" which causes most of us to forget the events of our childhood in later years.

We cannot dismiss offhand the possibility that many of those who suffered such malnutrition continued to have a carry-forward effect that led them to "acquire" a greater need for vitamins than would have existed without such malnutrition.

This possibility may also explain a curious contradiction in nutritional writings today. On one side is the view that a "good" diet, or a "balanced" diet, is all that is needed for good health. And it is pointed out that commonly available foods should make this possible for most Americans. Yet many seem to be puzzled that malnourishment is widespread, even among the affluent.

At this stage in our knowledge, we cannot discard the

possibility that such malnutrition—and much of our poor public health—has its roots in the past, in the Great Depression.

None of this can minimize the importance of food and proper vitamin supplements today. *If anything, as we have seen, such past malnutrition is likely to increase the need at present for high-level vitamin supplementation.*

Furthermore poor *current* eating habits can only add to the injury. As Linus Pauling has written:

> Many of the more affluent Americans also are suffering from a dietary deficiency. A specialist in nutrition once chided me for writing that many Americans would have improved mental health if they ingested more vitamins; he said that most Americans have enough money to buy food that provides their vitamin requirements. I replied that affluent people might have enough money to buy this good vitamin-high food, and still they might fail to spend it this way. Cola drinks, potato chips, and hamburgers do not constitute a good diet.

More than that. Many of us ate such junk foods in great abundance when we were teenagers. Too often in later years we repay this legacy by failing memory, weakening eyesight, poor or rotting teeth, and a host of other *known consequences* of poor childhood or teenage nutrition. Other consequences, only suspected as yet, may even add to the health importance of high-level vitamin regimens. None of us can relive his or her childhood and growing years. But we *can* shore up aging enzymes and restimulate flagging powers with compensatory vitamins.

CHAPTER 10:

Biochemical Individuality and the Biochemical Rights of Individuals

Many adults, who once as children were ready drinkers of milk, in their later years become unable to take this food without distress. Painful abdominal cramps are often the signs of an inability to digest the distinctive sugar found in milk (lactose). Up to 10 percent of Caucasians, a much larger percentage of Negroes, and many Orientals are so affected. In fact, one study of three sugar-digesting enzymes among 100 healthy adults showed a variation of ten to twenty times or more, in the levels of these internal secretions.

Another example of biochemical individuality was first reported at the mid-1973 American Medical Association meetings in New York. Allergist Ben F. Feingold of the California Kaiser-Permanente Medical Center described recent work with 25 hyperkinetic schoolchildren. Hyperkinesis means excessive motion, and sufferers from this behavioral disorder are jumpy, hyperactive, unable to concentrate or learn.

One 7-year-old in the study was described by Dr. Feingold: "When he was home, he stomped around, slamming the doors and kicking the walls, and even charging oncoming cars with his bike." Many of the children had a history of allergies, most had normal or high IQ's, and all had been eating large quantities of processed foods.

Dr. Feingold and his colleagues removed all foods with artificial flavors and colors from the youngsters' diets. Marked improvement was noted for fifteen of the twenty-five patients within just a few weeks. The 7-year-old mentioned above was reported as settled down, doing well at school, and no longer disruptive at home. But breaking the dietary regimen led almost immediately to a return of the hyperkinetic behavior. "We can turn these kids on and off at will, just by regulating their diet," Dr. Feingold noted. But he wondered about the practicality of keeping children on such restricted regimens since about 90 percent of processed foods contain artificial flavors and colors —including most children's favorites, such as hot dogs, soft drinks, and ice cream.

Dr. Robert Meiers of the Stanford Medical School has pioneered in treating "end-of-the-line" psychotic patients, those with whom every other treatment method has failed. Some of his patients were taken off drugs and fasted on nothing but water under close hospital supervision. "After fasting," he said, "they graduate to a raw vegetable diet, avoiding all animal food including dairy products and eggs, and avoiding grain. We permit raw fruit, vegetables, seeds and nuts as we slowly look for allergies."

The food items are restored one by one. Dr. Meiers noted: "We have run into some people who can't handle apples—one became psychotic again, one acutely paranoid, and one depressed."

Note that such individualistic responses to food elements (even to the minute trace amounts of artificial flavors and colors affecting hyperkinesis) can have pronounced behavioral (or "mental") manifestations as well as so-called physical ones. These responses, and many others, are merely recent striking examples of the well-known biochemical variability among different human beings. Every physician is well aware of this variability because he or she has seen differing reactions to the same drugs among different patients. Antibiotics or analgesics that one patient will tolerate well can cause grave illness in another or even (in rare cases) bring death.

In recent years it has become well established that clinically important diseases may be due to individual metabolic or digestive quirks. These may be present and manifest at birth. For example, phenylketonuria, called PKU, is a disease that accounts for about 5 percent of all retardation cases now in mental institutions. Today we know that PKU is due to an inborn inability to metabolize the common food element phenylalanine, an amino acid (protein) that causes permanent brain damage in the affected infants. Most newborn babies are now routinely screened for this defect, and PKU babies placed on a proper diet can have physical growth and mental functioning that is almost normal.

"Pyridoxine dependency" is another known genetic defect of recent discovery, this one directly related to vitamins. Without very large intakes of vitamin B6 (pyridoxine), the infants so afflicted suffer anemia, epilepticlike seizures, and mental retardation. A high-level pyridoxine regimen treats the disorder.

Biochemical Individuality

Such extreme variations of the internal chemistry that are present at birth make it likely that lesser variations, usually ignored medically, must also exist among most normally healthy people. Indeed, that we are all different chemically—except perhaps for identical twins—is obvious to the naked eye. Our differences of appearance and behavior must be mirrored in or caused by internal chemical differences.

Biochemical Individuality is the title of an important book by Professor Roger J. Williams, a distinguished scientist and leader in advocating the application of nutritional discoveries to medical problems. The concept began to become clear, he relates, in animal experiments. Researchers often use inbred strains of animals to minimize the differences of heredity, but such genetically similar animals still showed substantial biochemical differences.

Some inbred rats on identical diets excreted eleven times as much urinary phosphate as others . . . some voluntarily consumed consistently sixteen times as much sugar as others . . . *some appeared to need about forty times as much Vitamin A as others . . . some young guinea pigs required for good growth at least twenty times as much Vitamin C as others.* [Emphasis added.]

Vitamin needs in normally healthy human beings probably also vary just as widely, starting at birth and then continuing throughout life. Not all the scurvy-ridden sailors of the seventeenth and eighteenth centuries came down with the disorder simultaneously: Some were afflicted relatively soon, while others were resistant for many, many months longer, showing a great disparity in vitamin C needs.

A newborn baby, however, is not just the product of heredity. The infant has also just completed nine months of life *in utero,* and prenatal reactions to the mother's nutrition is part of the baby's chemistry. If the mother has been malnourished, for example, her children are likely to be born weaker, smaller, and stunted, possibly with a retardation in the development of the nerve cells, especially those in the brain. A 1973 study shows that alcoholism in the mother may have even more severe effects, as may various drugs or medications she takes during pregnancy.

Dr. A. Leonard Luhby and his colleagues at the New York Medical College examined 250 pregnant women for their status of the B vitamin folic acid. Over 20 percent were deficient, and Dr. Luhby stated this "could well constitute a public health problem of dimension we had not originally recognized," because such a deficiency could be passed on to the unborn child.

Life After Birth

As life progresses after birth, varying conditions of diet, activity, and stimulation also produce individual digestive and other chemical differences. Early diet, for example, influences the formation of the lining of the digestive tract and the nature of the digestive secretions as infancy and childhood progress. This in turn will probably have lifelong effect on the absorption into the bloodstream of nutrients from the food that is eaten. This absorption is known to vary greatly among normal individuals, affecting their dietary requirements. In addition, early food habits will have psychological effects, often creating eating habits that last a lifetime.

Another aspect of our individuality is the collection of bacteria within the digestive tract, known as the *intestinal flora*. Each of us does contain such a collection of mostly beneficial bacteria, varying from individual to individual. The intestinal flora relates importantly to our metabolism, aiding or inhibiting digestion, producing gas and other fecal material, and significantly producing (or consuming) vitamins. Vitamin K, in particular, which is vitally necessary for proper blood clotting, is produced in most healthy people by these intestinal bacteria, as are folic acid and other B vitamins.

Emotional factors are another cause of metabolic and digestive variations among individuals, even among laboratory animals. Loneliness or isolation has produced biochemical variations in laboratory rats, for example. Fear, stress, crowding, anxiety, tension—all affect the human internal chemistry, as do contentment, relaxation, and other states of calm and security.

Considering all the possible causes and types of biochemical individuality at different ages, and the differences already existing at birth, it is not surprising that chemical variations among apparently similar individuals are often not merely slight, about 25 to 50 percent, but major, ranging from 500 to 1,000 percent or higher.

The density of our bones, for example, is related to the body's utilization of calcium and vitamin D. Here X-ray testing has shown the variation among normal young men to be nearly sixfold. Thyroid glands will vary in weight from 8 to 50 gm, ovaries in normal young women from 2 to 10 gm, and so on. The shape and structure of many bodily organs and structures—muscles, tendons, ligaments, bones, etc.—will vary widely from person to person.

We can thus readily see evidences for individuality by:

- The gross anatomical variations among different people.
- The differences in blood and other body fluid composition.
- Differing levels of enzyme and endocrine activity.
- Variations in intestinal flora and excretion patterns.
- Different responses to drugs and chemicals administered.
- Varying patterns of illness and disease.

One could then not expect all persons to have the same nutritional needs, perhaps to be met by a single "balanced diet" or type of supplement.

The Biochemical Rights of Individuals

It is hard to escape the feeling that much of the above is obvious and hardly worth mentioning. That one man's meat is another's poison has always been the case and is not a controversial notion. Yet overlooking the obvious occurs all too frequently.

There is probably no such thing as a perfectly average individual when it comes to vitamin requirements. Each has his own distinctive personal needs, and a helpful vitamin regimen for one person may be too low in some vitamins for his brother—or wastefully high for his sister.

The authoritative *Heinz Handbook of Nutrition* notes that a typical person is not "one who has average requirements with respect to *all* essential nutrients and thus exhibits no unusually high or low needs. In the light of contemporary genetic and physiologic knowledge and the statistical interpretations thereof, the typical individual is more likely to be one who has average needs with respect to many essential nutrients but who also exhibits *some nutritional requirements for a few essential nutrients which are far from average.*" [Emphasis added.]

Thus, although few of us have special needs for *all* vitamins, *most* of us are likely to have special needs for *some* vitamins.

Our ways of determining these individualistic needs are still rudimentary. Much research remains to be done before we have procedures to tell how much of which nutrients each of us individually should have for optimum health.

In November, 1973, *Medical Counterpoint* called attention to "our massive ignorance regarding the clinical significance of the vitamins and the trace metals [which] is matched by our poor understanding of the role of most of them in biochemical processes."

Until our knowledge expands, it seems to make sense to maximize the chances for health by providing vitamins and trace minerals in the diet in abundant quantities, whenever this is possible and definitely known to be safe. Nothing less meets the natural desire of every person for optimum nutrition, even if that means vitamin (or mineral) quantities far above the average. This, we think, is the "biochemical right" of every individual—to be considered as an individual in his or her own chemistry and nutritional needs and to be permitted to have the foods (including supplements) to meet those needs.

CHAPTER 11:

Doctors, Drugs, and Vitamins

Vitamin researcher and Alabama physician Dr. E. Cheraskin recently wrote (in the foreword to Ruth Adams' helpful book, *The Complete Home Guide to All the Vitamins*) that he had received a telephone inquiry from a prominent man. His caller was uncertain whether he should take vitamins. This important personage had three attending physicians with different views. His ear-nose-throat specialist was insisting on a vitamin regimen. His internist discouraged vitamins on the grounds that he might get kidney stones. His urologist felt there need be no concern about kidney stones because he would merely harmlessly excrete excess vitamins.

Such variation of opinion among medical practitioners is not uncommon. Few physicians have had the opportunity to learn very much about nutrition and vitamins. Dr. Harvey Ross, a psychiatrist now applying vitamin and nutritional methods to his patients, has had to learn for himself. His statement may be typical: "I've gotten very interested in nutrition because it is so important. I don't remember anything about it in medical school except for a few lectures on the basic foods."

And Professor Jean Mayer has been widely quoted: "Our studies at Harvard among residents suggest that the average physician knows a little more about nutrition than the average secretary—unless the secretary has a weight problem, and then she probably knows more than the average physician."

The cause of this lack of knowledge is that medical schools have accorded nutrition almost no place in the curriculum. "Clinical nutrition is not even taught in most medical schools, and not really adequately done in any of them," said Professor Nevin S. Scrimshaw of M.I.T. in 1968.

Part of the reason for the lack of attention to nutrition and vitamins has been the great increase during the last thirty years in the number and type of drugs now used in medical practice.

"In 1940, the physician's 'black bag' was relatively small," points out Dr. George E. Burch, chairman of the Department of Medicine at Tulane, in a 1972 review of clinical medicine. "If it did bulge, it was apt to be filled with many carryovers from the 'weed and seed' days of medicine"—camphor, bromides, bile salts, and the like.

At that time there were no antibiotics for infections, nor antihypertensives for high blood pressure, tranquilizers, antidepressants, antihistamines, oral hypoglycemics, coricosteroids, radioisotopes—and there were no vaccines to prevent polio, German measles, mumps—no L-dopa for Parkinson's and related diseases, no isoproterenol for cardiogenic shock, no nonnarcotic pain relievers.

"All of these, and many more, are available to physicians today," he proudly notes. "There have been more significant drug discoveries and developments during the past 30 years than in the total history of man . . . [but] in the last decade, the rate of new drug development has seriously declined."

Some of this decline is due to more stringent legal requirements for testing for efficacy and safety; this testing can be lengthy and expensive. Another reason is that for many disorders, there are certain limitations in treatment by alien drugs. Most drugs tend to be merely palliative —that is, to alleviate symptoms rather than restore the patient's health.

Both drugs and vitamins should be necessary elements of the armamentarium of every physician. Both can provide great medical benefit. Both often work in relatively small quantities. Both are part of modern methods of treatment.

But drugs and vitamins do seem to work in different ways.

Drugs vs. Vitamins

Drugs are generally rapid in their action, while vitamins may be slow to take effect. A vitamin regimen often requires weeks or even months before a result is noticeable.

Many drugs have only a narrow and specific effectiveness, while vitamins are often systemic in their action, tending to influence the whole body. One single vitamin may affect many tissues and functionings—skin, hair, mouth conditions, muscle spasms, cardiac stress, ulcers, mental state, vitality, and so on.

Also, drugs are usually most effective when they are given alone, so that other powerful biochemical agents cannot interfere with their functioning. Vitamins, on the other hand, seem to work best in combinations, especially those combinations (with minerals) that in total provide good or optimal nutrition.

Professor Williams likens the physician giving a drug to an athletic coach working with a single track performer —runner, high jumper, discus thrower. Here, the sports achievement depends on this athlete's performance alone. By contrast, a vitamin is compared to a football player who needs a team working with him to function. What can a coach do with a star quarterback and no football team? asks Professor Williams, as he makes a case for a "complete" approach to nutrition in his persuasive book *Nutrition Against Disease.*

Another significant difference between vitamins and drugs relates to toxicity and side effects.

Drugs are generally foreign, alien substances, not nor-

mally found in the body. As a result, most drugs—even
ordinary household nonprescription drugs, called patent
medicines or over-the-counter (OTC) drugs—have a surprising toxicity, far above that of vitamins. For example, a
commonly used famous OTC cough medicine was withdrawn from the market in 1973 after the discovery that it
had caused more than a dozen deaths!

*By contrast, we don't believe there has ever been one
fatality due to excessive vitamins.*

Aspirin, our most commonly used drug, is another case
in point. Hundreds of childhood deaths are reported annually in the United States alone due to accidental aspirin
poisonings, but this distressing news usually does not
make the newspapers. Aspirin is a known toxic substance:
The lethal dose is about 0.2 gm to 0.3 gm per pound of body
weight or 20 gm to 30 gm for an adult (60 to 90 common
aspirin tablets), and a lesser amount for children. Indeed,
aspirin is the most common single poison used by suicides,
second only to the several barbiturates.

Analgesic pain killers such as aspirin are only one type
of dangerous drug. Adverse effects often also follow the
use of antacids, those bubbly solutions we take by the ton
for upset stomachs. Antihistamines have caused many
fatalities. Freely sold nose drops and cough medicines
often produce severe side effects.

And remember, these are all nonprescription, over-the-
counter drugs. Prescription drugs are usually notably more
toxic. *More than 30,000 Americans die each year from adverse reactions to antibiotics, it was disclosed in hearings
in Congress in 1974. And hundreds of thousands perish
from infections by drug-resistant bacteria, caused by over-
use of drugs.*

Vitamins, on the other hand, are foods. This means that
they are normally found in the body. They are natural to it.
In the course of time, vitamins are consumed as they are
used by the body in its regular processes.

Except for vitamins A and D, most vitamins are virtually

harmless in any quantity to persons of average health, and few have side effects of significance. The water-soluble B vitamins and vitamin C on rare occasions and with some people can produce minor symptoms of distress if taken in very large quantities. But even these are only slight digestive effects (stomach upsets, laxative action) and are less than would be felt after ingesting similar amounts of common substances, such as table salt.

Vitamins A and D can produce damage if wildly excessive doses are taken, such as one hundred times the amounts of vitamin D in our proposed regimens. But even these dangers are usually greatly exaggerated. One medium serving of ordinary nutritious beef or calf liver, which nobody fears to eat because of its vitamin A content, contains more than twice as much vitamin A as our "high-level" regimens. No permanent damage has ever resulted from vitamin A overdose, even to people who took absurdly high doses for long periods of time, since the excess vitamin was gradually used up by the body.

The central fact is that, by comparison to medicinal drugs, vitamins are exceptionally safe. The body requires them continually for good health and uses them up as a normal function.

Drugs may be fast, powerful, and specific, but as alien elements in the body, their presence is always a disturbance to the normal metabolic processes. Overdose damage is the rule rather than the exception, and it can often be most severe. Also, such drugs are unlikely to have the long-term preventive and restorative effects of vitamins.

Drugs and Malnutrition

In addition to their side effects, it is now also becoming clear that many drugs "share the potential for causing malnutrition," as Dr. Daphne A. Roe of Cornell University announced in 1973. According to her research, there are four ways in which drugs alien to the body can set the stage for nutritional deficiencies. They can depress the appetite, impair the body's ability to absorb nutrients, cause a loss of minerals and vitamins, or interfere with the mechanisms for using vitamins.

Amphetamines, for example, used as diet pills for the overweight and in the treatment of hyperactive children, can suppress appetites to the point of malnutrition, especially for such trace nutrients as vitamins and minerals. Other drugs used in the treatment of gout, psoriasis, high cholesterol levels, and blood disorders can inhibit the absorption of the fat-soluble vitamins A, D, and K. Even a common laxative (phenolphthalein) that is widely used can cause such malabsorption, Dr. Roe has pointed out.

Oral contraceptives—the birth control pill—can cause deficiencies of vitamins D, C, and B6.

At present, the FDA requires that the advertising of prescription drugs include a thorough description of their side effects and other dangers. (The layman, in fact, would be generally horrified to read the small print in the pharmaceutical companies' advertisements in professional medical and dental journals because the possible side effects of most drugs are so severe.) "Over-the-counter" drugs requiring no prescription—such as aspirin, antacids, cough medicines, and the like—have fewer, but still often frightening, potential side effects.

But none of these drugs are sold with any indication to consumer, patient, or even physician that they can induce vitamin deficiencies. Here is a matter that has been overlooked by the Food and Drug Administration, with potential for mass damage to health.

Why Vitamins Act Slowly

If vitamins are so fundamental compared to drugs, why do they frequently act so slowly, often taking weeks or months for their effectiveness to become evident?

Consider the following example, described by the late

noted nutritionist Adelle Davis. A woman whose face was disfigured with hundreds of unsightly warts came to her for advice. A highly nutritious diet with an exceptionally large vitamin A supplementation was suggested. The woman adopted this regimen, but months passed with no results. Both began to lose heart. Then abruptly, after four months had gone by, all of the many warts disappeared within one week.

Of course, there is no *proof* that the vitamin A regimen was responsible. Readers with warts are cautioned that this is just one case, warts are generally not removed by vitamin A, and excessive amounts of vitamin A can, of course, be harmful. But lack of this vitamin—and of several others as well—is known to induce many types of skin conditions.

Whatever the curative agent, it is clear that new tissue growth had to take place. Such regeneration cannot be immediate because *growth takes time.*

Similarly, inside the body many conditions may involve the structure of the internal tissues and organs. Hormones, for example, are the chemical regulators of many bodily functions. Circulating in the bloodstream in tiny amounts, hormones control our metabolism, bodily growth, sexual functionings, often our moods and emotions, and so on.

Hormones are produced by the endocrine glands—the adrenals, the pituitary, the thyroid, and others. The patterns of hormonal secretion will depend on the cells and tissues of these endocrine glands. How well or poorly these cells and tissues are nourished will in turn affect their growth and functioning. If additional tissue is to be created in these glands, time must also pass for this new growth to occur.

Also, it is likely that the linings of our blood vessels may develop lesions which then may become thickened with the waxy fat substance called cholesterol, a state known as *atherosclerosis.* This was believed once to be found only in the aged but is now known to be astonishingly widespread. Autopsies on young soldiers killed in combat showed 72 percent had such cholesterol deposits, and even children and infants now often have signs of this fatty degeneration of their blood vessels.

When the arteries are so thickened internally by deposits, there is a greater likelihood that a small blood clot or a fragment of such a deposit itself, drifting in the bloodstream, can "plug" the artery. If this occurs in an artery supplying the heart muscle, it can cause a heart attack. If this takes place in the brain, a stroke may result. Or, over time, these fatty deposits can become impregnated with minerals, especially calcium, which is "hardening of the arteries," a stage of *arteriosclerosis*. Senile dementia and other serious consequences result from such calcification of the arteries.

But what of the effects on vitality, strength, and general health of atherosclerosis *before* such grave conditions arise? This has not been measured, but it is a medical fact that reduced circulation can lower vitality and energy.

Imagine a pipe that is thickened inside, so its internal radius is reduced. The flow of fluid through that pipe must also be reduced. In fact, there is a law of hydrodynamics called Poiseuille's Law that says that the volume of a flow through a rigid tube goes down sharply when the internal radius is reduced. For example, if the radius is reduced by *one-half*, the flow is reduced to *one-sixteenth*. A relatively small change in the vessel size produces a relatively large change in the flow.

Thus the general effect of atherosclerosis on total health could be one of slow weakness and fatigue in total physical and mental functioning (the brain definitely needs an adequate blood supply), with no obvious clinical signs. Nobody knows the extent of this effect on general health.

Cholesterol is found in many naturally occurring foods, such as animal fats, eggs, milk; it is also produced within the human body by many tissues, especially the liver. Cholesterol must be so produced because it is a necessary part of the body's manufacture of vital elements, including sex hormones and vitamin D, and is an integral part of every living cell. When cholesterol is not present in the diet, the liver can and will manufacture it in quantity. In fact, it is believed that even with a high-cholesterol diet, the liver regularly produces more cholesterol than is eaten.

The medical problem is clear. Cholesterol (and similar fats) are necessary in the body. But how can such substances be prevented from being deposited on the walls of the blood vessels? And, if deposited, how can they be removed?

As we will see later, not only do several vitamins have the power to reduce the levels of cholesterol (and other potentially damaging fats) circulating in the bloodstream, but the latest and most startling research, reported as recently as November, 1973, has shown that a high-level regimen of the B vitamin *folic acid* has actually reduced the lesions of atherosclerosis in human patients.

Such healing, however, takes time. The removal of already-deposited cholesterol, if it occurs internally, would also take time—several weeks or months—because such a process involves a physical alteration within the body.

These may be some of the reasons why vitamin regimens, unlike drugs, often need time for their full effects to take place and be evident as an improvement in health. But the turnaround in the body chemistry that vitamins create can usually be felt in weeks, and then it continues, slowly increasing toward vitality and strength.

We began this chapter noting that nutrition has been a stepchild in the medical curriculum and that many physicians have overlooked its importance in creating states of good health. Happily, this situation is changing rapidly. The new vitamin discoveries and the modern concern for preventive medicine are becoming more widely known and increasingly influential, especially among physicians. And, more and more, the importance of nutrition is also being realized by others.

Knowing the facts rather than the fancies of cellular and total-body nutrition may be our best hope for a restored national health. The maintenance of cellular nutrition is essential to the normal performance of physical and mental tasks, as well as to longevity. A finely tuned instrument is a joy to hear. A finely peforming well-nourished living cell in response to the demands of life can also be a source of joy to the body that contains it. As the cells make up the body, the individuals make up the nation. Knowledge and good practice cannot be left to physicians alone: The individual must also learn and do. Toward that end, we now turn to specific information about vitamins, minerals, and other nutrients, as a prelude to the regimens themselves.

CHAPTER 12:

Vitamins from A to P

The Fat-Soluble Vitamins

The four fat-soluble vitamins, A, D, E, and K, measured in International Units (IU's), often need the presence of fats and minerals, and sometimes one another, to be absorbed properly into the body from the digestive tract. To compensate for periods of low vitamin intake, these can also partly be stored up within the body. Mineral oil (which is not a nutrient) can dissolve these vitamins and flush them from the intestinal tract. Unlike the water-soluble vitamins, excess intake of vitamins A and D can sometimes be troublesome, though the greater danger for most people is inadequate intake.

VITAMIN A

Found in fish (especially the liver oils), and also in butter and the liver fats of various animals, this vitamin can also be manufactured by the body from the "carotene" in yellow vegetables, such as carrots and yellow sweet potatoes, and also in very green vegetables (spinach, turnip, dandelion, and beet greens). But the vegetable sources are often overrated, for as the Food and Nutrition Board notes: "the availability of carotenes in foods as sources of Vitamin A for humans is low and extremely variable."

There are several reasons for this. In raw carrots, for

example, the carotene is within the indigestible cell walls, and only 1 percent or less may enter the body. Also, the efficiency of the conversion of carotenes to vitamin A may be as low as one-sixth or less.

Liver, eggs, whole (but not skim) milk, fortified butter, and margarine are the best dietary sources of vitamin A.

The first distinctive effect of a lack of vitamin A is usually night blindness, which is an inability to see under conditions of darkness. The eyes may take a long time to adapt to dim light in theaters or outdoors at night after leaving a lighted area. Dry skin, itchy eyes, and skin rashes may also accompany the night blindness. Modern interior lighting conditions, especially strong office lights, may cause the body to use up its stored vitamin A at a rapid rate, producing complexion problems due to inadequate vitamin A. Other deficiency signs include further eye disorders (including corneal ulcers), dry and brittle hair, poor growth in young animals, loss of appetite and weight, sterility, and increased susceptibility to infections.

In 1966 Dr. Umberto Saffiotti (Associate Scientific Director for Carcinogenesis of the National Cancer Institute) made front-page news when he reported on experiments with hamsters and lung cancer.

When smoke containing carcinogenic agents (similar to those found in smog and cigarette smoke) was blown into the lungs of the hamsters, cancers were induced in these animals. But when vitamin A was added to their diet, the development of these cancers was retarded to a significant extent. Of course, this does not mean that vitamin A is a "cure" for cancer but merely that it helped prevent the cancers from arising.

This was believed to be due to this vitamin's necessity for the integrity and efficiency of the epithelial cells and mucous membranes—*i.e.*, those that line the respiratory passages. Well-functioning cells here can, by their mucus flow and cilia action (tiny hairs that brush away damaging matter), help protect the body against air-borne cancer-producing particles, just as they help prevent bacteria and viruses from obtaining a foothold and thereby protect against infectious disease.

In addition, vitamin A is stored in the liver, which has as one of its chief functions the purification of the blood. Foreign poisons often collect there to be detoxified, and it is believed that vitamin A plays an important role in dealing with such deleterious substances as pesticide and fertilizer residues, industrial poisons such as carbon tetrachloride, and other toxic drugs.

The U.S. Recommended Daily Allowance is 5,000 IU's for adults, 6,000 IU's for pregnant women, and 8,000 IU's for nursing women, but daily doses of 100,000 IU's have often been administered to adults for months or years without ill effect. Signs of vitamin A overdose (nausea, irritability, aching bones, headaches, hair loss, increased pressure in the cranium, which may be mistaken for a brain tumor) disappear rapidly when the intake of the vitamin is reduced.

In all of the history of medicine there are only about two dozen recorded cases of persons who took too much vitamin A and suffered any distress. Although vitamin A overdose is to be avoided, there is no cause for avoidance of those intakes that can be beneficial. In fact, Professor Jean Mayer calls insufficient vitamin A "one of the main causes of blindness" in America.

Even though normal cooking and heating do not destroy the vitamin, borderline deficiencies are believed widespread. This has been verified by autopsies in which the vitamin A content of the liver has been examined and found wanting. These deficiencies can arise from inadequate intake of the vitamin itself or of other nutrients needed for its absorption or utilization: vitamin E, protein, the B vitamin choline, fats, and zinc. (Vitamin A therapy for patients with obvious deficiencies has sometimes been found to be ineffective unless supplementary zinc is also provided.)

Despite its potency (4,000 IU's of vitamin A is only 2.4 mg), vitamin A is one of four nutrients that careful surveys by the Department of Agriculture over thirty years have consistently shown to be in short supply in the American diet. (The others are vitamin C, calcium, and iron.) Diabetes, malabsorption, a poor diet, the depletion of bodily vitamin A reserves by pollutants or exposure to strong lights, can all contribute to a lowered vitamin A store within the body and thus to increased susceptibility to infection and other disease, skin and vision problems, and so on.

VITAMIN D

This is the "sunshine" vitamin, so called because sunlight acting on the oils of the skin can produce it and then it is absorbed into the body (if the oils have not been washed away just before or just after sunning). After a suntan is established, no further vitamin D is believed created. The only naturally occurring food sources are fish-liver oils; thus, cod-liver oil has been the traditional dietary supplement for infants and growing children who need the vitamin most, since without it they suffer the severe skeletal malformations called rickets.

The value of vitamin D for adults was first authenticated by studies among Moslem women whose seclusion and covering garments kept sunlight from their skin. After many years of deficiency, they developed troublesome bone difficulties. Today we know the bone weaknesses of the elderly—fragile and easily broken bones, bones that will not readily heal after being broken—can often be traced to insufficiencies of vitamin D or calcium.

Current smog conditions in industrial countries often severely reduce the vitamin D-producing sunshine rays from reaching the surface of the earth. Today we irradiate most milk to provide a source of vitamin D in the diet, though night workers, nuns and others whose clothing or customs keep them fron sunlight, and dark-skinned persons living in northern climates or smog-covered cities are especially advised to take supplements of this vitamin if they do not regularly drink vitamin D-fortified milk. Children who do not drink a full quart of such milk daily certainly need such supplements.

Many years before Columbus, the Norsemen, led by Eric the Red, established a colony in the frigid area of Greenland. Skeletal remains show that the women of the colony developed pelvic bone deformities that prevented them from childbearing, so the outpost eventually died out. Apparently the Norsemen would not eat the fish bones (for calcium and phosphorus) or the fish livers (for vitamin D) that the Eskimos do. Insufficient sunlight in that northern region led to the bone deformities.

One theory of the distribution of the human races over the surface of the earth emphasizes the role of sunshine and vitamin D. Overdoses of vitamin D can be toxic, beginning with general depression and diarrhea, and then leading to abnormal calcium deposits in the soft tissues, the blood vessel walls, liver, lungs, kidney, and stomach. Sunstroke may also be related to excessive intake of vitamin D.

The theory is that under primitive circumstances, the dark-skinned equatorial peoples could not thrive under conditions farther north where the sunlight was weaker because there they would get insufficient vitamin D. Similarly, the lighter-skinned northern peoples would suffer vitamin D overdoses under tropical sunshine conditions. One or the other of these groups, moving into the opposite region, would gradually, over millions of years of evolution, lose its portion of "wrong-skinned" people. The environment would "select," or winnow out, the proper-hued group for survival and cause the others to vanish, in the Darwinian survival of the fittest.

The darker skin of the peoples on the Indian subcontinent and the native Australians is explained by this theory, as well as that of the Africans—and also the very light, almost transparent coloring of some of the peoples of northern Scandinavia. All of these differences are attributed to a balance between vitamin D need and vitamin D overdose.

About 400 IU's is the officially recommended daily amount of vitamin D for infants, children, growing teenagers, and pregnant and lactating women. Since vitamin D deficiency can also cause constipation, muscular and nervous weaknesses, cramps, and other complaints in adults, our vitamin regimens call for higher amounts, especially for teenagers, and also for older persons whose bones may be weak. The Food and Nutrition Board notes that, beyond infancy, "there is no evidence that intakes of the order of 2,000 to 3,000/day produce hypercalcemia," and even these safe amounts are well above those we recommend.

In fact, the most up-to-date standard medical references, such as Louis S. Goodman and A. Gilman's *A Pharmacological Basis of Therapeutics* (Fourth Edition, 1970) and *The Merck Index* (Twelfth Edition, 1972), suggest that harm in adults can only result from intakes of vitamin D on the order of 100,000 to 150,000 IU daily for many months. Thus no adult need fear vitamin D overdose from our proposed vitamin regimens of 800 to 1,200 IU daily, which are about one-hundredth of those amounts. For this vitamin, 1,000 IU is the same as 25 micrograms.

In mid-1974, Dr. Claus Christiansen and associates of the Glostrup Hospital in Denmark reported that vitamin D therapy helped control epileptic seizures among hospitalized patients. The study lasted eighty-four days and included twenty-three patients, all of whom had been on anticonvulsant drug therapy for periods of three to seventeen years, and this was continued during the trial. "The results should provide ammunition for the pro side in the long-standing debate over the effectiveness of prophylactic vitamin D therapy for epileptics," noted *Medical World News* (June 14, 1974).

VITAMIN E

The technical name for this vitamin is "tocopherol," coming from *tokos,* the Greek word for "childbirth," *pherein* meaning "bring forth," and *-ol* for "oil"—the "oil of fertility." This name was given because vitamin E was first discovered by researchers who found its absence would lead to reproductive failure in rats (by resorption of the fetus).

Vitamin E has become something of a fad in recent years, as news has spread of its necessity for proper muscle functioning, of its anticlotting and circulation-improving abilities, of its beneficial effects on the lungs and heart (which is a muscle), and on aging—and, above all, of its relation to sexuality.

Actually, vitamin E is a vital if only recently popular nutrient which is unlikely by itself to serve as an aphrodisiac or potency restorer. Its absence does, however, prevent reproduction in many animals and does cause anemia and muscular weaknesses in man and monkeys.

One of the best sources of vitamin E is fresh whole-grain wheat products, and it is also found in many vegetable oils (corn, soybean, safflower oils, but not olive oil), especially when the oils have not been subjected to high heat treatment. Best are the "cold-pressed" or "expeller-pressed" oils available in health food shops or health sections in the supermarket. There is also some vitamin E in liver, beans and peas, butter, eggs, and leafy green vegetables. Despite this apparent abundance of sources, there is much evidence that many Americans do not get enough vitamin E.

For proper absorption of vitamin E from the intestinal tract, the presence of fats and vitamin A is believed necessary, and this absorption is inhibited by the mineral iron (whose salts can destroy vitamin E if excessive iron-containing foods are eaten with it simultaneously).

Chemically, vitamin E prevents the deterioration or rancidity of fats and oils by acting as an antioxidant—that is, by preventing premature oxidation of these fat compounds. Diets that are high in polyunsaturated oils, now a current fad, thus increase the body's needs for additional vitamin E.

Azo dyes are man-made organic compounds, many of which are used as artificial coloring agents in food. Others are known to produce cancerous tumors in animals. A number of animal experiments have now shown that the number of cancers induced by azo dyes is reduced when vitamin E is also added to the diet. Also, transplanted tumors do not grow as rapidly (if they grow at all) when ample vitamin E is given, and the growth of cancer cells in blood plasma decreases in the presence of vitamin E.

Dr. Otto Warburg was one of the most famous of twentieth-century chemists. Shortly before his recent death he wrote a book, in 1967, called *The Prime Cause and Prevention of Cancer.* His thesis was that cancer derives from an oxygen deprivation at the cellular level; cells so deprived have their metabolism turned askew—they then turn "wild," cancerous. Vitamin E's antioxidant properties reduce the need of cells for oxygen, and this may explain its cancer-retarding effects in these animal experiments.

Other notoriety has come to vitamin E from the work of the Canadian physicians and heart specialists, Dr. Evan Shute and Dr. Wilfred E. Shute, formerly brothers in a common practice. In a 1972 book, *Vitamin E for Ailing and Healthy Hearts,* Dr. Wilfred E. Shute and co-author Harold J. Taub note that despite a substantial drop in animal-fat consumption in recent decades,

> heart-disease deaths have doubled since 1945, far outstripping the growth in population and amounting today to more than one million deaths a year in the United States. By far the major cause of such deaths is coronary thrombosis [*i.e.*, a blood clot stopping up the coronary artery that

supplies the heart muscle with oxygen and nutrients], which occurs frequently even when there is no atherosclerosis.

Is there, then, a more rational explanation than the animal fat-atherosclerosis theory to explain why a disease entity that did not occur prior to 1910 has become a greater ravager of human life than any plague recorded in history?

Vitamin E is also a known "antithrombin"—circulating in the blood, it can dissolve blood clots and prevent such clots from forming unnecessarily. Also, it improves circulation, thus benefiting muscular functioning. (Athletes on vitamin E regimens often show less fatigue after exertion and can be capable of improved performance—and for this reason, vitamin E supplements have often been used by Olympic and other athletes.) The relevance of this vitamin to heart disease is clear because the heart is a muscular organ.

Dr. Shute believes that for coronary thrombosis, "there is an explanation so simple that it would automatically be suspect had its truth not already been demonstrated in clinical practice of more than 20 years involving many thousands of patients."

When the modern type of white flour began to be produced, "the diet of Western man lost its only significant source of Vitamin E. Flour milling underwent this great change around the turn of the century, and it became general around 1910. The amount of Vitamin E in the diet was greatly reduced, and with the loss of this natural antithrombin, coronary thrombosis appeared on the scene."

This theory gains some support from the recollections of the late famed heart specialist Dr. Paul Dudley White, who wrote in his own book, *Heart Disease:*

> ... when I graduated from medical school in 1911, I had never heard of coronary thrombosis, which is one of the chief threats to life in the United States and Canada

today—an astonishing development in one's own lifetime!
There can be no doubt but that coronary heart disease has
reached epidemic proportions in the United States. . . .
The truth is, an ever-increasing number of young men are
being struck down before the age of 40. . . .

A high-level vitamin E regimen is the major part of the
Shute treatment of heart disease (with special precautions
taken for high blood pressure and rheumatic heart cases)
and is recommended by the doctors as a preventive measure. Controversy and debate surround this matter because
not all heart specialists have had similar results, but the
possibilities of widespread but unrecognized vitamin E
deficiencies are very real. Up to 1973, the Food and Drug
Administration by an admitted blunder never established a
Minimum Daily Requirement for vitamin E, so most vitamin supplements and fortified foods completely omitted
this vitamin. And while the Food and Nutrition Board in
1968 listed a daily Recommended Dietary Allowance of 30
IU's, one careful study of food from supermarket shelves
suggested that the average American was getting less than
8 units each day.

Recall Dr. Fitch's experiment with the vitamin E-
deprived rhesus monkeys, in which there were no signs
of deficiency for up to thirty months, following which an
abrupt and devastating anemia was invariably fatal. The
normal life span of this monkey can range between twenty
and twenty-five years, about one-fourth or one-third that of
man. On the human scale, it is possible that vitamin E
deficiencies or low-reserve states could exist for a decade
or longer without being noticed. The effects on general
circulation and overall physical strength resulting from
such a long-term deficiency could be profound, even for
those who do not have heart attacks or strokes owing to
blood clots.

Vitamin E is one of the few nutrients that do not well
survive long storage when frozen, so as frozen foods have

increased in the diet, vitamin E intake has declined further for most of us.

This should be considered in light of the fact that there are many reports of the therapeutic benefits of vitamin E for various circulatory complaints (varicose veins, vascular degenerations arising from diabetes, etc.), for external use as a treatment for burns, and for the general signs of aging.

The physician Dr. Christopher Cook (of the Association of Life Insurance Medical Directors) has written, for example: "I believe that Vitamin E slows down the process of aging, so that taking it in sufficient daily amounts can possibly make a person of 60 look, act, feel, *seem*, and *be* more like a person of 50, or a person of 70 look, act, feel, seem, and be more like a person of, say, 60."

Except for sufferers from high blood pressure and rheumatic heart conditions, vitamin E is believed safe in any quantities. The Food and Drug Administration states that it is "harmless when taken for prolonged periods." The Food and Nutrition Board notes: "toxicity symptoms have not been reported even at intakes of 800 I.U. per kilogram of body weight daily for five months." (This would be a total daily intake of 56,000 IU for a 154-pound man—an unheard-of quantity.)

But those with rheumatic heart conditions should not take supplementary vitamin E except under medical supervision. High blood pressure cases should begin with small doses and have their blood pressure carefully monitored as the dosage increases. (Since vitamin E improves the efficiency of the heart, it can drive the blood pressure up in hypertensive patients, though it does not have this effect on others.) Rheumatic heart fever sufferers have an imbalance between the two sides of the heart. Large vitamin E doses can increase the imbalance, worsening the patient's condition.

The *alpha-tocopherol* fraction of the tocopherol compounds has the most vitamin E activity. For this vitamin, 1 IU is the same as 1 mg.

VITAMIN K

A Danish researcher found this vitamin when investigating hemorrhages among chickens and so named it because the Danish word for the clotting of the blood is *koagulation*.

Vitamin K is indeed necessary for proper human blood coagulation, or clotting. Without it, internal bleeding and hemorrhages may occur. Although some vitamin K is contained in foods (leafy green vegetables, corn, tomatoes, strawberries, potatoes, eggs, wheat bran and germ), the main source for most people is believed to be the bacteria in their intestines. These friendly and beneficial organisms, called the *intestinal flora*, can manufacture vitamin K, following which, in the presence of fat and bile, it can be absorbed into the bloodstream.

If these bacteria are destroyed, as sometimes happens after treatment by antibiotics, they should be restored. Eating yogurt is one quick and healthful way to do this. (The intestinal flora also manufacture B vitamins, especially folic acid.)

Vitamin K may be administered medically when there is insufficient blood-clotting ability, especially among infants, but this is rarely found among adults. When it does occur, professional medical care is needed immediately. Vitamin K is *not* included among our proposed vitamin regimens.

The Water-Soluble Vitamins

The B vitamins and vitamin C, because they dissolve in water, tend to be absorbed more readily by the body than the fat-soluble ones. Then they circulate throughout the entire body, where they are involved in the basic processes of metabolism at the cellular level.

These are the vitamins that, with the appropriate minerals, make up the "wick" in which the fuels of the body are burned for energy, and which also provide the spark for the processes that constantly create new cells and tissues. The body does not store these vitamins to any great extent and always needs a fresh supply. Because they dissolve in water, excess amounts are readily excreted in the urine, and for healthy people, these are safe in nearly any quantities. No medical harm is possible from overdoses.

Many of these vitamins work together in different stages of complex chemical reactions. When one vitamin is missing, the whole reaction must come to a halt. Thus the initial symptoms of vitamin deficiency are often similar, especially for the B vitamins: depression, nervousness, skin and mouth disorders, eye complaints, diarrhea, general debility, and so on. More serious or prolonged deficiency can lead to heart and abdominal pains, hallucinations, hemorrhaging, paralysis—and even death.

Many of the B vitamins are found together in natural foods, such as whole grains, nuts, and liver. Others are variously found in meats, fruits and vegetables, and dairy products. Vitamin C is most abundant in green and yellow peppers, citrus fruits, other fresh vegetation, and liver.

These vitamins are not as stable as the fat-soluble ones. The heat of cooking, storage, exposure to air or light, soaking or prolonged cooking in water can destroy them. So can many forms of food processing, and alkaline solutions, such as those of baking soda.

VITAMIN C

This vitamin, whose chemical name is *ascorbic acid,* has been a center of controversy in recent years. It has long been known that a prolonged lack of vitamin C produces the mortal disease of scurvy—and lesser insufficiencies often lead to bleeding gums, blood vessel fragility (producing many black-and-blue marks on the skin), bone and teeth weaknesses in growing children, anemia, general debility, and an increased susceptibility to infections.

The latest research verifies that vitamin C in large amounts does protect us against colds and minor illnesses, promotes the healing of wounds and injuries, and may also sharpen mental abilities.

Soldiers under the extreme stress and tension of battlefield combat have drastically reduced vitamin C reserves in their bodies, indicating this vitamin has important antistress properties. Research with animals tends to verify this significant finding.

In addition, this vitamin aids in the absorption of iron into the body, helps overcome foreign poisons, has been useful in treating schizophrenia and ulcers, has helped cataract patients and those with back complaints, and demonstrated a host of other health benefits.

Vitamin C is used in every living cell in the fundamental metabolic processes of life and also has special functions in the white blood cells (which fight infection) and in the manufacture of collagen, a binding substance that holds all cells and the bones together. Further, there is growing evidence that vitamin C protects the circulatory system against damaging fatty deposits.

Several surveys show that vitamin C, which is not abundant in grains or most cooked animal foods (except liver), is not consumed in sufficient amounts by large segments of the population. The elderly, who often avoid fresh fruits and vegetables, are especially prone to vitamin C deficiencies.

In its pure form, vitamin C is a white crystalline powder that dissolves readily in water to form a colorless solution, slightly acid but not unpleasant to the taste. In addition to its use as a dietary supplement, it has also been used to keep fresh fruit and vegetables from darkening when serving, canning, or freezing.

In some persons, the intestinal flora apparently have the power to destroy ingested vitamin C unless there is sugar present for them to feed on. Thus vitamin C is best taken after a meal or snack, especially one containing fruit.

The *Journal of the National Cancer Institute* has reported an experiment that showed that transplanted tumors in guinea pigs grew less rapidly when vitamin C was abundantly supplied. In man the cancer-producing nitrosamines (from fertilizer residues or nitrate and nitrite food preservatives) are believed to be combated by vitamin C.

Writing of his own experiments with guinea pigs in *Science* in February, 1972, Dr. Emil Ginter of the Institute of Human Nutrition Research in Bratislava, Czechoslovakia, noted:

> The relationship of cholesterol in [blood] serum and Vitamin C intake has been demonstrated in humans. If our conclusions are applicable to the human organism, we shall probably find that latent hypovitaminosis C [*i.e.*, insufficient vitamin C, but too mild a deficiency to be observable] can cause hypercholesterolemia [excessive cholesterol], and that it may also play a role in the pathenogenesis of atherosclerosis.

In other words, undetectable vitamin C deficiencies are likely to cause high cholesterol levels, which in turn may lead to atherosclerosis. To gauge the importance of such research, recall both our high rate of atherosclerosis and that vitamin C is one of the four nutrients found most wanting in the American diet by the U.S. Department of Agriculture.

Several books have been written about the many protective powers of vitamin C, and Americans everywhere are realizing that the official recommended allowances (up to 60 mg for adults) are woefully inadequate for the best health. Even television entertainers have publicly announced their own greater health via vitamin C; Merv Griffin, for example, recently told his audience that he takes 2,500 mg daily and has not had a cold in five years.

Vitamin C can often prevent or counteract chemical

poisonings from such toxic agents as the metals lead and arsenic, and other poisons such as carbon monoxide, benzene, bromides, and severe overdoses of aspirin. Insect bites and plant toxins (poison ivy, poison oak) can also be detoxified by vitamin C.

Dr. P. K. Dey of the University College of Science in Calcutta, India, for example, gave selected groups of mice doses of the severe poison strychnine, some with vitamin C and some without it. All of the mice who got no vitamin C died of convulsions. Those mice also given one gram of vitamin C per kilogram of body weight survived, some with few or no convulsions.

Japanese quail were the experimental animals used by M. R. Spivey Fox and Bert E. Fry, Jr., of the Department of Nutrition of the Food and Drug Administration to test the effects of vitamin C on cadmium poisoning. Cadmium, a fertilizer contaminant, produces anemia together with low iron concentrations in the liver among these birds. But when vitamin C was added to the diet, no anemia or other adverse effects were noted.

Dr. Fred R. Klenner of North Carolina, author of *The Key to Good Health: Vitamin C*, uses this vitamin extensively in his practice with patients, both by injection and orally. "I frequently give as much as 150 grams intravenously in 24 hours for such things as monoxide poisoning and barbiturate poisoning," he notes, citing excellent results, and adds that it is also useful against bacterial and viral infections, and for burns when applied as a spray.

Thus vitamin C can help the body overcome foreign poisons that result from air, water, and food pollution. In addition, it is a known agent against personal stress, which can rapidly deplete the body's small reserves of vitamin C. Interestingly, there are even cases where it seems to substitute for other water-soluble vitamins that may be lacking in the body.

In May, 1974, *Medical Tribune* informed American physicians of the work of Dr. B. D. Rawal and his colleagues at the University of Queensland, who reported on the anti-bacterial action of this vitamin. "Indeed, when administered together with [antibiotics] . . . to cystic fibrosis patients . . . there was a marked reduction in [hostile bacterial] organisms, a decrease in spectum, and improved well-being."

VITAMIN P

Is there a vitamin P? This is one of the controversial issues in current nutritional and health thinking. If so, it is found among a group of substances called the "bioflavonoids" (rutin, narigin, hesperidin) occurring in the pulp and white rind of citrus fruits and in extracts of red pepper. These are believed to augment the effects of vitamin C, promote healing, and benefit the circulatory system. Studies in the Soviet Union, Germany, and the United States show they may also exert protective effects against excessive blood clotting and arterial degeneration.

For example, one such study by R. C. Robbins (published in 1967 in the *Journal of Atherosclerosis Research*) used 260 rats divided into 20 groups. Some were fed diets that would promote internal blood clotting; others got diets that would favor atherosclerosis. With bioflavonoids added, 18 of the 20 groups showed an average increase in survival time under their adverse diets.

Because we are unaware of any certified sources of vitamin P supplementation by pills or tablets, we will recommend another way for you to include the vitamin P substances in your nutritional regimen.

THE B VITAMINS

There are 11 B vitamins that are widely accepted (others may also exist) and that are included in our vitamin regimens. These are:

B₁—Thiamin

B₂—Riboflavin

B3—Niacin (two chemical forms: nicotinic acid and nicotinamide, the latter also often called niacinamide)
B6—Pyridoxine
B12
Biotin
Choline
Folic Acid (also called Folacin)
Inositol
PABA (Para-aminobenzoic Acid)
Pantothenic Acid

THIAMIN—VITAMIN B1. This was the first discovered and remains the best known of the B vitamins. Its most severe deficiency causes the mortal disease called beriberi, whose symptoms are weakness, paralysis, heart pains, and cardiac failure. Lesser deficiencies are known to reduce the efficiency of the brain and central nervous system. Added thiamin has even been found to improve learning and intelligence in several experiments.

The Food and Nutrition Board makes special note of the fact that "older persons use thiamin less efficiently" and consequently must be more alert to maintain an adequate dietary intake.

Thiamin is a relatively cheap vitamin to manufacture commercially, so it is every food processor's favorite added vitamin to boost the sales of baked goods, breakfast cereals, snack foods, and the like. It is one of the three vitamins added by law to bleached white flour (the others are riboflavin and niacin, which are also inexpensive).

Although nearly every one of us eats enough thiamin to avoid marked deficiencies, it is questionable whether we receive enough for the best functioning of our nervous systems and for optimal mental health. One study of food in England shows that on the average we only take in about one-fourth the thiamin consumed by English peasants five hundred years ago.

RIBOFLAVIN—VITAMIN B2. Cracks around the mouth and lips, frequent occurrence of bloodshot eyes, and a purplish tongue are clinical signs of a riboflavin deficiency. An increased sensitivity to light, together with a need for bright lighting for proper vision, are other manifestations of a lack of this vitamin.

Riboflavin is a yellow pigment in pure form. It is found in beef and chicken liver, nuts, beans, milk and milk products, and so on. It is unusual in that it can be destroyed by light, as frequently used to happen when milk in clear bottles sat on the morning doorstep for hours and hours. Today much riboflavin in milk is destroyed by the light that is used to create vitamin D in milk.

Some relief of cataracts has been attributed to vitamin B2 therapy, and its lack causes anemia, burning sensations in the hands and feet, loss of hair and weight, and so on. These are common signs of malnutrition at the cellular level, for this vitamin is needed for the proper biochemical functioning of every living cell.

In addition, riboflavin aids the body in the absorption of iron from the digestive tract, and animal experiments show it has special cancer-inhibiting properties.

NIACIN—VITAMIN B3. This is the third B vitamin used to "enrich" white flour and bakery products. It comes in two forms, *nicotinic acid* and *nicotinamide* (also called *niacinamide*). Nicotinic acid has an immediate effect when ingested in substantial quantities that can often be felt within a few minutes as a "flushing," or warming of the skin in the extremities, especially the hands and forearms. Some find this momentarily uncomfortable, while others do not mind, stating it tells them "the vitamin is working." The effect soon wears off and tends not to appear at all after some weeks of high niacin intake. Administration of nicotinamide, on the other hand, has been reported to cause some depressions among mental patients on niacin therapy.

An extreme deficiency of niacin causes the mortal disease called pellagra, with mental symptoms (hallucinations, dementia), skin rashes, and diarrhea. Lesser deficiencies give rise to depression, irritability, insomnia, backaches, headaches, and so on. Niacin plays a major role in the new methods of orthomolecular psychiatry now being used to treat schizophrenics and autistic children, and also in maintaining healthful nonexcessive fat levels in the bloodstream. Cow's milk and dairy products contain very little niacin.

PYRIDOXINE—VITAMIN B6. Essential for the metabolism of every amino acid protein, pyridoxine is especially important to help overcome the nausea and toxemia of pregnancy, some adverse effects of birth control pills, and is otherwise beneficially related to skin conditions among both sexes, convulsive and epileptic states, heart conditions, ulcers, anemia, rheumatism, menstrual and menopausal disorders, and possibly diabetes.

Bananas are a good source of pyridoxine, as well as raw meat, as in steak tartare. The heat of cooking is especially destructive of this vitamin.

Dr. John M. Ellis, author with James Presley of the 1973 book *Vitamin B6: The Doctor's Report,* believes pyridoxine deficiency is the most widespread deficiency disease in the United States, causing many types of muscle and nerve pains, and unnecessary swellings, and may be linked to rheumatism.

For normal adults, the official U.S. Recommended Daily Dietary Allowance is only 2 mg (2.5 mg for pregnant or lactating women), yet the prestigious Food and Nutrition Board notes that in observations of large human population groups in Burma and Malaya, "estimated daily intakes of between 1 and 2 mg were associated with considerable evidence of biochemical aberrations." This seems to be cutting it very close, especially since pyridoxine needs go up with protein intake and Americans eat more protein than the Asians observed. Dr. Ellis recommends a *minimum* supplementation of 50 mg for adults (100–300 mg for pregnant or lactating women).

In infants, a pyridoxine deficiency can be manifested by extreme convulsions. In adults, anemia can be the first sign, followed by difficulties with the tendons and ligaments, especially in the hands, and swellings there and elsewhere.

New research from London's St. Mary's Hospital reported in 1973 shows that half of the women who become depressed while taking birth control pills can be benefited by additional pyridoxine, and the British medical journal *Lancet* now strongly recommends such vitamin therapy for all women on the "pill."

Pyridoxine is another of the B vitamins that reduces the level of free cholesterol circulating in the bloodstream and thus may aid in combating atherosclerosis.

VITAMIN B_{12}. This vitamin is virtually absent from all vegetable food sources. Only meat or animal products can be a food supply of vitamin B_{12}, which is essential for the normal functioning of all cells, but particularly for those of the bone marrow, the nervous system, and the gastrointestinal tract.

A lack of vitamin B_{12} (or folic acid) causes pernicious anemia, which manifests both blood weaknesses and an irreversible neurological degeneration leading to paralysis and blindness. "Vegetans," as vegetarians are called who will eat no meat products (such as milk and eggs which contain vitamin B_{12}), have been especially prone to this crippling malady.

The Food and Nutrition Board notes that "Evidence indicates that the ability to absorb Vitamin B_{12} may decrease with age," so older persons should take special care to insure an adequate supply in their diet or by supplements. The body's needs for vitamin B_{12} are measured in micrograms, or millionths of a gram.

Reporting on new research, *Medical Counterpoint* in December, 1973, noted:

> When Vitamin B12 is given to patients with pernicious anemia, there is customarily a rapid improvement in mental state and in the feeling of well-being, all occurring days before the onset of any hematological [blood] change. Accordingly, the vitamin has been given for the symptom of fatigue alone in patients who have no clinical evidence of B12 deficiency. The reported studies have all been defective until recently.

The new research was conducted very carefully by two investigators in Great Britain, Dr. F. R. Ellis and Dr. S. Nasser, working at Kingston and Long Grove Group Hospitals, and reported in the 1973 *British Journal of Nutrition* in an article entitled "A Pilot Study of Vitamin B12 in the Treatment of Tiredness."

The doctors began by soliciting private physicians and hospital staff members for patients (or staff) who had inexplicable feelings of fatigue. Twenty-nine subjects, male and female, were gathered and completed the trial. All were given complete physicals and examined for vitamin B12 deficiency periodically. Heavy smokers were excluded. Half the patients got twice weekly injections of 5 mg of vitamin B12 for two weeks. The other half got a similar-appearing but inert (placebo) injection. Neither the patients nor those who examined them (or gave the injections) knew which was which—that is, the trial was "double blind"—to avoid the effects of suggestion or wishful thinking. Then there was a two-week resting period (no injections), followed by a switch: those who had earlier gotten the vitamin got the placebo (fake injection), and vice versa, all still under double-blind conditions.

The patients filled out questionnaires each day about their appetite, mood, energy, ability to sleep, and general feelings of well-being. In summarizing this research paper, the American journal for physicians, *Medical Counterpoint*, noted: *"Statistically significant improvement in mood and the feeling of well-being occurred in the patients given the vitamin in contrast to the placebo. The effects persisted for at least four weeks."* None of the patients had any evidence of a vitamin B_{12} deficiency before the experiment.

The patients who started with the vitamin treatment continued to have increased well-being throughout the two-week resting period and the following two weeks of placebo injections, and also maintained high vitamin B_{12} blood levels during this entire four-week period. Those who began with the placebo reported no improvement until the fifth week (when they began receiving the vitamin).

Let us note that those getting the vitamin were receiving 10 mg (10,000 mcg) weekly by injection. The new (1973) U.S. Recommended Daily Allowance of this vitamin is only 6 mcg daily, or 42 mcg a week. Since injections are usually about four times more potent than vitamins taken orally (because of absorption difficulties), the experiment's subjects were receiving the equivalent of about 40,000 oral mcg or more weekly—or approximately *one thousand times* the recommended daily allowance.

More recently, University of Virginia researchers reported the discovery that this vitamin exerts a strong protection among certain microorganisms against viruses. Whether this anti-viral action also occurs in humans remains to be seen.

BIOTIN. This vitamin is found in many foods—liver, peanuts, beans, eggs, oysters, as well as whole grains—and milder deficiency states (believed rare) produce lassitude, lack of appetite, depression, muscle pains, and skin changes. Severe biotin deprivation produces heart conditions and paralysis.

Biotin deficiency states are uncommon, and because vitamin manufacturers are today unable to produce sufficient biotin, the Food and Drug Administration has delayed until 1977 its order requiring that more than tiny amounts of biotin must be present in supplements containing this vitamin. (Most supplements that do have biotin contain just a minuscule fraction of the amount believed needed each day.)

Biotin, needed for the metabolism of fats, can be destroyed within the body by a substance in raw egg white, which is how deficiencies in experiments have been induced in human volunteers.

CHOLINE. The Food and Nutrition Board notes that: "dietary choline protects against poor growth, fatty liver development, and renal [kidney] damage in many experimental animals, and against perosis, or slipped tendon, in the fowl. Also, it has been reported to protect against abnormalities in pregnancy and lactation in the rat and mouse; anemia in the guinea pig, rat, and dog; cardiovascular disease in the rat; and muscular weakness in the guinea pig and rabbit." In addition, the absence of choline causes high blood pressure in some animals, while added choline improves fertility in others.

Choline, found in whole grains, liver, and vegetable foods, is important in the human body's manufacture of thyroid hormones, in the functioning of the nervous system, and to prevent cirrhosis of the liver. It has been beneficially used with heart attack survivors and to treat viral hepatitis, a liver infection. Choline also inhibits cancer growth in animals. Together with inositol, it is used in the internal manufacture of lecithin in the human body, which is believed to help remove damaging cholesterol from the walls of arteries and to dissolve it in the bloodstream.

FOLIC ACID. Also called *folacin*, this vitamin derives its name from the same root as the word "foliage," because it is found in spinach and other green-leaved vegetation. A lack of folic acid produces gastrointestinal upsets, diarrhea, and more seriously, pernicious anemia, which has both blood and neurological manifestations and is caused by a lack of *either* folic acid or vitamin B_{12}.

The Food and Nutrition Board notes: "A folacin deficiency may arise from four main causes: inadequate dietary intake, impaired absorption, excessive demands by tissues of the body, and metabolic derangements."

It takes about five months for pernicious anemia to develop when folic acid is deficient in the body. If folic acid is present but vitamin B_{12} is absent, then only the neurological manifestations of pernicious anemia appear and though these are irreversibly damaging, without the accompanying blood signs, they are hard to diagnose. For this reason, until 1973, the Food and Drug Administration limited the amount of folic acid that could be present in dietary supplements to only 0.1 mg per day without prescription.

The newer regulations, possibly the result of much agitation by nutrition groups, raises this amount to 0.8 mg in supplements labeled "for pregnant or lactating women," and 0.4 mg in those for adults and children over the age of four years. Though a step in the right direction, this is but a small step. *Prescription* dosages are also limited by the FDA to no more than 1.0 mg per tablet by the new 1973 rules, even though folic acid is safe in almost any amounts in the body.

Ironically, a few months after the announcement of the new FDA regulations, Dr. Kurt A. Oster reported (in *Medical Counterpoint*, November, 1973) on his clinical work with elderly diabetics who had visible atherosclerotic lesions and with hyperuricemic (gout-prone) patients. Dosages of folic acid between 40 and 80 mg were used with notable success in both types of cases. We will later describe his work—which moves folic acid to first place among inhibitors of atherosclerosis—in more detail because of its great potential importance. Let us here merely note that the official daily allowance of folic acid is only 0.4 mg for adults, which is one-hundredth or less than these therapeutic quantities. If the new FDA regulations continue to stand, even physicians treating patients by prescription will be unable to provide proper medication, unless the patient is to swallow 80 pills daily or they ask a colleague in Canada to supply them with higher potency tablets.

INOSITOL. This B vitamin is not recognized as essential to human health by the Food and Nutrition Board. Perhaps this is because inositol can be partly manufactured in the body from other nutrients. In the normal state the human body does contain more inositol than any other vitamin except niacin.

Supplementary inositol has been reported to help overcome baldness, constipation, eczema and dermatitis, and poor appetite.

In *The Complete Home Guide to All the Vitamins*, Ruth Adams notes: "It is noteworthy that, among the organ meats, inositol is very abundant in heart muscle. It is axiomatic that those organs in which vitamins or minerals are stored have special need for those nutrients."

In addition, inositol is an important constituent of lecithin, which the body also manufactures and which is believed to protect against cardiovascular disease by lowering blood cholesterol (and triglyceride) levels.

PABA (PARA-AMINOBENZOIC ACID). This is another disputed vitamin, not being recognized as such by the Food and Nutrition Board but being listed as a vitamin in several standard medical references. The sulfa drugs work as antibiotics by counteracting PABA in bacteria, so the side effects of these drugs in man—nervousness, hallucinations, depression, digestive upsets—are actually symptoms of PABA deficiency.

PABA has been shown as beneficial to many skin conditions and is also reported as preventing the graying of hair. In some cases it is even credited with a restoration of hair color after grayness has occurred.

As an external ointment, PABA offers the maximum protection against sunburn so far encountered among all chemical agents tested, and also protects against the aging and skin cancers that excessive exposure to sunlight can cause. This was discovered in 1969.

PANTOTHENIC ACID. This B vitamin is not disputed, being recognized as essential by the Food and Nutrition Board, which calls it "of the highest biological importance" and notes that deficiencies produce

> biochemical defects [that] may exist undetected for a time, but they eventually manifest themselves as symptoms and signs of tissue failure. In animals, this may be indicated by infertility, abortion, small litter size . . . the growth rate of young animals is retarded. . . .
>
> In man, deficiencies are slow to develop . . . [but produce] . . . headaches, malaise, nausea, and occasional vomiting accompanied by flatulence and abdominal cramping . . . cramping of the muscles of the legs . . . and impairment of motor coordination . . . [and] loss of antibody production. Subjects deficient in either pantothenic acid or pyridoxine formed antibodies sluggishly, but men deficient in both failed completely to form antibodies. . . .

Antibodies, of course, protect us against hostile bacteria and viruses, so these two B vitamins, pantothenic acid and pyridoxine, are thus vital for the body's defenses against infectious diseases. Pantothenic acid is also important as a protective agent against stress, and experiments we will describe later show that it may also help to increase longevity. Interestingly, this vitamin is a major constituent of the honey bee's "royal jelly."

New evidence from England now links the crippling and

mysterious malady of arthritis to a pantothenic acid deficiency. The biochemist E. C. Barton-Wright stated, in April 1974, "I am not claiming I have discovered a permanent cure for arthritis. What I do claim is that we have discovered the *cause*, the method of *control* and the method of *prevention*." (Emphasis added.) His answer? Pantothenic acid!

OTHER B VITAMINS. Other possible B vitamins are B_{14}, which Dr. Neil Solomon of the Johns Hopkins University Medical School cites in his recent excellent book *The Truth About Weight Control* as acting in the bone marrow to produce new blood cells, and B_{15} (pangamic acid), believed related to muscular activity, and B_{16}. The Russians have been particular leaders in investigating these new vitamins and demonstrating their therapeutic and restorative properties.

CHAPTER 13:

Minerals from
C to Z

Minerals, in many ways similar to vitamins, differ by being *inorganic* chemicals. This means that living organisms cannot create them. Plants must extract minerals from the earth, and animals must extract them from their food.

The human body does not consume, or "burn up," minerals in quite the same way that it does organic (carbon-containing) compounds, but it does have a continuing need for minerals. Calcium and phosphorus make up the actual structural material of our bones and teeth and play a role in the functioning of the soft tissues as well. Sodium and potassium are needed for nerve transmission and the proper excretion of wastes. Many minerals are regularly and necessarily excreted from the body in urine and sweat.

The basic life processes of individual cells through the whole body do require many minerals, in a manner similar to their need for vitamins. In fact, very often vitamins and minerals are known to work together—calcium and vitamin D, selenium and vitamin E, magnesium and vitamin B6 (pyridoxine), and so on.

As with many vitamins, a shortage of a mineral may be reflected by distinctive clinical signs, such as those of rickets, goiter, weaknesses in blood clotting, anemia, and others. Lesser deficiencies can give rise to tension, insomnia, fatigue, depression, irritability, skin and hair problems, and so on. Cases of defects in muscular contractility, poor neurological responses, and heart dysfunction have responded to supplemental minerals. All of these manifestations can be indications of cellular malnutrition, similar to the case of vitamins.

Many minerals—iron, copper, iodine, chromium, selenium, manganese, zinc—are needed in small amounts, measured in milligrams, micrograms, or smaller quantities. Some of these can be quite toxic if excesses are ingested. Others—calcium, phosphorus, magnesium, sodium, potassium, chloride—are required in larger amounts, and these are not toxic but often require a "balance" among them for optimal health.

One problem with minerals in nutrition is that while they are not destroyed by the heat of cooking or by storage, many minerals are only poorly absorbed from the digestive tract. The absorption of calcium, for example, is ordinarily so inefficient that 60 to 80 percent of ingested calcium usually passes through the body and is lost in the feces. (Excess fats in the diet further reduce calcium absorption, while vitamin D and milk sugar enhance it.)

Similarly, only about 10 percent of ingested iron is normally absorbed. The iron in leafy vegetables such as spinach is particularly unavailable (medicinal iron is absorbed better than food iron). Also, only 4 to 8 percent of the chromium we eat is absorbed, and similar fractions of several other minerals that are eaten are actually used.

However, by mysterious mechanisms not yet understood, in cases of deficiency the body can often increase its absorption of some selected minerals.

There is a constant turnover of the mineral composition of the body, even some of that of the bones, so a fresh supply of minerals in the diet is a constant necessity for good health.

Calcium

The Mexican peasant gets his calcium from the limestone on which his corn is pounded. The Eskimo gets his from the fish bones he gnaws. But the major sources for Americans are milk and milk products, since much of the natural calcium in wheat and sugar is refined away in their processing.

Pregnant and lactating women have a special need for calcium, and it is also especially needed for bone development or maintenance by infants, growing children, and older persons. A lack of calcium often contributes to the particular bone problems of the elderly—the easily broken bones, and the hips and limbs that heal so slowly and painfully.

Osteoporosis is a thinning or weakening of the bones by loss of calcium. The Food and Nutrition Board notes: "There is a relatively high prevalence of this disease in older persons in the United States, the incidence being higher in females than in males and apparently higher in whites than negroes. In many osteoporotic individuals, *calcium supplements have induced calcium retention and improved bone density ... an inadequate calcium intake over a period of years may contribute to the occurrence of this disease.*" [Emphasis added.]

But calcium has other bodily functions as well. It is necessary for proper blood clotting, muscular activity, and the functioning of the nervous system.

Calcium has powers as a nerve tranquilizer to overcome irritability and grouchiness, as a calming and sedative agent to help insomniacs sleep better, and as a painkiller. Calcium injections have also been used for the pains of pleurisy and migraine, and in my own [Dr. Rosenberg's] case of broken ribs, intravenous calcium was most effective. Oral calcium (often with vitamin D) is used for labor pains, the discomforts of visits to the dentist, arthritis, muscular aches, cramps, menopausal disorders, and so on. The value at bedtime of the proverbial warm glass of milk to help one get to sleep, for example, is attributed to its calcium content.

Large amounts of sugars and other carbohydrates in the diet can prevent the absorption of calcium, as can bicarbonate of soda and excesses of phosphorus, with which calcium is in "balance" in the body. After the first year of infancy, the amounts of calcium needed daily range from 0.8 to 1.4 gm or more. Unless toxic levels of vitamin D are taken simultaneously, there are no dangers from an excess of calcium in the diet.

Two investigators reported in 1967 that calcium "may retard increases in cholesterol and other lipids [fats] in the blood and exert a protective action against the development of arteriosclerosis." Verification comes from additional experiments by others which showed that increasing calcium in the diet did lower cholesterol and triglycerides (another damaging fat) in the blood of young people. Further, extra calcium in the diets of rats prevented the damaging contaminant cadmium from producing high blood pressure, fats in the bloodstream, and heart abnormalities.

Since the refining of flour and sugar have made milk and dairy products the only major potential dietary sources of calcium in the modern diet, and since many adults drink little milk, it is not surprising that calcium is included among the four "most missing nutrients" by the Department of Agriculture, and is in short supply in many of our bodies. But we cannot recommend whole milk (or skim milk) as a dietary source of calcium for adults for two reasons. First, many adults have a "lactose intolerance," which causes gastric distress after drinking milk. Second, and perhaps more significant, is the work of Dr. Kurt A. Oster of Bridgeport, Connecticut, which indicts homogenized milk as a major cause of atherosclerosis and other heart and circulatory diseases. We will describe the startling implications of Dr. Oster's work in a later chapter. Mineral supplements—to be described later—are thus desirable especially for the elderly, to insure adequate dietary calcium. Calcium "overdose" is impossible.

Phosphorus

The other major constituent of our teeth and bones, phosphorus, is generally well supplied in the American diet—perhaps too well, since phosphorus is common in meats, seafood, eggs, dairy products, many vegetables, and so on. An excess of phosphorus can cause calcium losses in the urine, and this is believed to be one cause of calcium deficiencies.

Phosphorus is important for kidney and nerve functioning, the production of hormones and lecithin, and metabolism at the cellular level. Most of the brain is made up of fats which have been combined chemically with phosphorus.

Iron

This is the mineral needed for hemoglobin, the vital red-blood-cell pigment that carries oxygen to all our body cells and removes carbon dioxide from them. Iron is also in many enzymes produced by the body and is especially important for muscle functioning.

Meats and eggs are the best dietary sources of iron (cow's milk and dairy products contain little), and there are some vegetable sources: whole grains, grapes and raisins, apricots, molasses, dates, dried beans and peas, and greens. But these are often inadequate, especially for women in the childbearing ages who are menstruating, pregnant, or lactating. Even the Food and Nutrition Board notes that the stated objective of its Recommended Daily

Allowances, to meet good health needs among essentially all individuals in the general population, *"cannot be met by ordinary food products in respect to iron."*

A lack of iron causes anemia, which can lead to general debility, depression, dizziness, and other symptoms of bodily weakness. Iron-deficiency anemia is common among children and women who do not take dietary iron supplements. Adults need 10 to 20 mg of iron daily to maintain their iron stores, which the Food and Nutrition Board states are "greatly reduced or absent . . . in two-thirds of menstruating women and in the majority of pregnant women. It is impractical to supply these needs with ordinary food, and iron supplementation is required."

In the past, when people ate more vitamin C (which aids in the absorption of iron) and more whole-grain foods, the iron intake from food was much higher than it is today.

Magnesium

Magnesium is related to calcium and phosphorus, and is also necessary for the bones, teeth, and soft tissues. But about 80 percent of the magnesium is lost when whole grains are refined to make white flour, and none is returned in the "enrichment" process. The polishing of rice removes a similar fraction. Dr. Neil Solomon notes:

> until recently, magnesium deficiencies were not given the respect which we now know they deserve . . . the more protein food you eat, the more magnesium you need. Too much sugar in the diet can also lower magnesium absorption. Excessive use of alcohol can deplete magnesium stores. . . . A word of caution to persons habitually using diuretics to control fluid retention: along with the water loss there is also a loss of magnesium.

Dr. John Prutting, president of the Foundation for the Advancement of Medical Knowledge, says: "People who habitually start the evening meal with Martinis, a cheese appetizer, and go on to steak or hamburger with potatoes and dessert lower their magnesium level dangerously."

And he adds, "undernourished hospitalized patients given large doses of Vitamin B1 and other vitamins by injection remained deficient in those same vitamins until magnesium was added to the injections; then the vitamin deficiencies cleared."

The importance of a magnesium deficiency may be gauged from Professor Roger J. Williams' evaluation; he asserts: "Mild magnesium deficiency may be widespread, and a disastrous deficiency may not be uncommon among those suffering from heart attacks."

And in its official publication, "Recommended Dietary Allowances," the Food and Nutrition Board states: "Animals fed moderately low levels of magnesium, *sufficient to allow normal growth and prevent all gross signs of deficiency,* often develop calcified lesions of the soft tissues and increased susceptibility to the atherogenic effects of cholesterol feeding." [Emphasis added.]

In other words, an otherwise undetectable, or subclinical, magnesium deficiency can still lead to atherosclerosis and harmful mineral deposits in the soft tissues.

The need for magnesium is about half that of the need for calcium, a proportion found in the naturally occurring mineral *dolomite,* often used as a supplement. Since a great magnesium excess can cause the signs of calcium deficiency (lethargy, weakness, slow heartbeat, and, in the extremes, coma), this balanced supplement is one of the best ways to augment the magnesium component of the diet.

In the days when Epsom salts were a common household remedy, magnesium deficiencies may have been much less since Epsom salts is the chemical magnesium sulphate.

Iodine

Without iodine, the thyroid gland in the neck expands, causing the often irreversible condition called goiter.

Iodine is necessary for the manufacture of the thyroid hormones. Since iodine is mostly found in seafood, at one time goiter was endemic in the American Midwest and other places where the soil is poor in iodine and seafood was rarely eaten.

The iodization of salt was introduced to overcome this deficiency. Many countries of the world require that all table salt be so augmented, but the United States does not. Although it is inexpensive to treat salt this way, and iodized salt generally costs no more than unsupplemented salt, many regions of the country seem to prefer the unaugmented salt. The result is many iodine deficiencies, and even cases of goiter, in several areas of the United States, even today. Restaurants and other commercial food preparers also often use un-iodized salt, so that constant restaurant eaters who avoid seafood may also receive insufficient iodine.

The amount of iodine is very low in cereal grains, legumes, and other vegetables. Meat and dairy products are only good sources when the animals have been grazed on iodine-rich grasses or given similar rations. But there is no way of telling whether the meat, eggs, milk, and cheeses available to you contain any iodine at all.

The amounts needed are measured in micrograms, from about 100 to 150 daily for adults, or more. Larger amounts, up to 2,000 mcg, have been taken daily for years by children under medical supervision without any ill effect. The Food and Drug Administration now limits iodine in supplements to 300 mcg, which many nutritionists feel may be inadequate. Adelle Davis, for example, reported that she took a 100-mg (100,000 mcg) dosage each week "on a prescription written by a kindly dentist." When she could not get this weekly iodine supplement, one drop of medicinal antiseptic iodine solution daily in a glass of water was her substitute.

Sodium, Potassium, Chloride

According to the majority of health authorities, most of us get too much sodium and chloride (ions) at present, because these are the ingredients of table salt, sodium chloride. There are many unanswered questions about these minerals.

These are necessary minerals, so the questions revolve around how much is desirable. High blood pressure, or hypertension, has been induced in animals by an excess of sodium, but many efforts have failed to duplicate this condition in man.

On the other hand, the Japanese who eat a very high salt diet do suffer as a group from a high incidence of hypertension and strokes. A relatively salt-free diet has been one method of high blood pressure treatment for many years, but is not notably successful.

Nonetheless, sodium is a necessary nutrient for every cell and the body, especially needed when hot weather conditions cause profuse sweating. When more than four quarts of liquid are drunk daily, salt supplementation is recommended, if many salty foods are not otherwise eaten. Otherwise, heat prostration and sunstroke may result.

Sodium and potassium are in balance in the normal body, potassium inside the cells and sodium just outside them, together facilitating the flow of materials into and out of each cell.

Potassium deficiencies can cause low blood sugar, gas and indigestion, muscular weakness or paralysis, and degeneration of the heart and similar consequences. Potassium is widely distributed in foods (meats, fish, fruits, vegetables, nuts, grains, some dairy products), but since the absolute amount of potassium is not as important as its relation to sodium, those who eat many salted foods should seek to augment their potassium intake. Potassium chloride salt substitutes mixed with ordinary table salt may be one convenient way to do this. A daily glass of orange juice can also do much to boost potassium intake.

Chromium, Cobalt, Copper, Manganese, Molybdenum, Selenium, and Zinc

These are additional minerals, some known to be necessary for good health in small amounts, and others merely suspected to be essential.

Without *copper,* for example, anemia and bone disease occur in man, and animals show defects in pigmentation, structure of hair or wool, reproductive failure, cardiovascular lesions, etc. (A daily intake of 2 milligrams appears to be needed for adults.)

Chromium and *cobalt* are more questionable. These are trace or microelements in human nutrition, needed (if at all) in billionths of a gram or lesser quantities.

Manganese is known to be essential, needed for normal bone structure. *Molybdenum* and *selenium* are believed to work in enzyme systems, the latter with vitamin E, which it can sometimes replace when needed. *Zinc* is recognized as necessary for both animals and man, and zinc therapy has been beneficial in cases of anemia, vitamin A lack, short stature due to glandular defects, liver and spleen conditions, skin sores, and sex gland problems, when tissue levels of zinc and zinc intakes were low.

The tiny, or trace, amounts needed of these minerals can nevertheless be essential for good health. Dr. Leon Hopkins, a trace mineral specialist with the Department of Agriculture, writes: "Trace element deficiencies do exist in large numbers of people in this country . . . We cannot assume that animals, including man, are obtaining adequate amounts of the various trace elements for optimum health from plant foods. Soil depletion, increased processing of foods and feeds, and changing eating patterns are forcing us to change our concepts in mineral nutrition."

Dr. Henry Schroeder and his colleagues at Dartmouth

Medical School and Brattleboro Memorial Hospital agree, noting that for minerals generally, "the enriched residues from the refined carbohydrates of wheat and sugar cane are fed to poultry and livestock, whereas human beings eat the depleted material. . . . The average American diet . . . is probably marginal, and in some cases, partly deficient in several essential micro-nutrients, especially . . . chromium, zinc, and possibly manganese."

Many minerals have variously been shown to be needed or protective in different ways. *Iron* inhibits cholesterol formation in the liver, as does *chromium. Selenium* aids in protecting our internal fats from oxidation. *Potassium* deficiency causes sudden death from heart lesions in animals. And so on.

In fact, one of the mystifying findings to heart disease investigators was the statistical discovery in the 1960's that cardiovascular mortality is generally lower in regions that have "hard" water. Soft water has fewer minerals and is more convenient for washing. But the minerals that make water "hard" seem to reduce heart attacks of all types. This is a further demonstration, if any were needed, as to the importance of adequate mineral intake to our health.

Mineral Supplements

If an individual's daily need for magnesium is 400 mg, of what value can a dietary supplement containing only 1 milligram of magnesium be? Similarly, calcium, which is needed in amounts of about 1 gram, is often found in supplements in quantities of only one-twentieth or less of this amount.

Minerals are continually being lost from the body in urine, sweat, and feces, and many minerals are not readily absorbed from the digestive tract. Knowing this, many persons have long taken mineral supplements. But many of these supplements have contained ridiculously low amounts of minerals, woefully inadequate. Unsuspecting buyers, unaware of the actual amounts needed daily, often believe that the mere mention of a mineral on a label means that the supplement does supply some substantial part of the body's daily needs for that mineral. And unscrupulous vitamin and health food manufacturers have been quick to take advantage of the gullible and unknowing.

Some of this may change for the better if the new 1973 Food and Drug Administration regulations (which we will describe later) take effect. These call for certain minimal amounts of "mandatory" minerals—calcium, phosphorus, iodine, iron, and magnesium—and of "optional" minerals as well—copper and zinc—when these are included. The amounts must be more than minuscule and thus actually be of some use to the body.

Even here, however, the permitted calcium and phosphorus can be at very low levels. In later pages we will tell how you may more securely provide an adequate mineral intake for yourself.

CHAPTER 14

The Building, Energy, and Roughage Foods

We have all heard of *proteins, carbohydrates,* and *fats,* but there are many misconceptions about these nutrients. And also about *roughage,* which is a special indigestible foodstuff, usually a technical form of carbohydrate.

Fats and carbohydrates are the energy foods, the fuels that keep the body (and mind) going. Proteins are the major building blocks of the body, though in a pinch they too can be used for energy. Roughage, not strictly speaking a nutrient at all, is nonetheless needed for the proper functioning of the digestive tract.

Protein

All the living cells of our soft tissues, the hair and nails, enzymes, hormones, the red blood cell pigment hemoglobin, and other body constituents are primarily made up of proteins, more than 1,000 of them. Proteins are large complex molecules containing nitrogen and are themselves made up of simpler compounds called *amino acids.*

There are 22 different amino acids that have been found in plants and animals, but the human body is believed to contain only 20 of them. These amino acids are linked together in chains of great molecular length and complexity to form the giant protein molecules.

When a protein food is eaten, the digestive juices break

it down into its component amino acids, which can then be recombined in the cells to build the tissues and other protein parts needed. Research has shown that only 8 amino acids, called the *essential amino acids,* are needed in the adult diet (infants need at least one additional amino acid for proper growth). From these 8, plus additional nitrogen, the body can create or synthesize the other amino acids it needs, and then the proteins themselves. A food that contains all of the 8 essential amino acids in roughly the right proportions is called a *complete* source of protein.

When such complete protein is lacking, a host of minor health complaints can ensue: chronic fatigue, falling hair, edema (swellings), skin wrinkles, irritability and grouchiness, increased susceptibility to infections, loss of sex drive, and other signs of accelerated aging. Even overweight can result because water may accumulate in the tissues under insufficient protein conditions.

We often tend to think of protein as being only in animal meats, fish, eggs, and dairy foods, and while these are good sources of complete proteins, they are not the only ones. Individual plant foods do not as a rule provide complete protein (soybeans are the best), but combinations of these can be just as nourishing and complete as animal meats and fish, especially when augmented by dairy products (which also contain the vital vitamin B12, lacking in all pure plant foods). The Latin American peasant often combines beans and corn in his diet, which together are a complete protein source. In India, rice can replace the corn. Elsewhere in the world, wheat and other grains, or nuts, are added to beans or milk or cheese, to augment the dietary protein in vegetarian societies or in those where meat, fish, and eggs are rare luxuries.

Some typical American foods that are thought to be the best sources of protein—steak and hamburgers, for example—are actually overrated. Red beefsteak, "choice" grade, is only about 17 percent protein—the rest is fat (25 percent), water (about 50 percent), and indigestible fiber. "Prime" beef has even more fat and less protein. Ounce for ounce, poultry and fish actually have more usable complete protein.

The average adult needs 65 gm or more of "good" protein each day for the best health. This is about the amount in 8 eggs, 6 glasses of milk, 7 ounces of lean hamburger, 9 ounces of sirloin steak, or 6 ounces of chicken breast or fish. But even in wealthy America, many people do not get the daily protein they need. "Perhaps surprisingly, even the affluent, sophisticated urbanite may suffer from protein-calorie malnutrition," asserts Dr. Neil Solomon, after examining the diets of typical businessmen and suburban housewives.

To be useful in the tissue building purpose of protein, all of the essential amino acids must together be present in the digestive tract *at the same time.* If any one of them is absent or eaten as soon as an hour or two later, the body seems to give up on creating protein. It cannot store the amino acids it has. Instead it burns the incomplete collection for energy. In fact, if there are insufficient carbohydrates or fats in the diet or in the body's reserve store of energy (fat), then ingested protein will be burned for energy. If dietary proteins are also lacking, then internal organs will start to be consumed because the energy needs take precedence—this condition is actual starvation.

Without vitamins, proteins cannot be utilized properly. Vitamin B6 in particular is needed for protein metabolism. Interestingly, there is enough of this vitamin present in raw animal meat for its metabolism, but the heat of cooking destroys much of it. Thus an outside source of this vitamin is needed if the best use is to be made of the meat protein that is eaten. Primitive man who ate his meat raw had no need for supplemental vitamins!

Fats

Fats are needed in the diet to help absorb the fat-soluble vitamins and then to "transport" them within the body. Fats are so necessary that when they are absent, the body will convert carbohydrates to fat. Without dietary fats, water may also be retained within the tissues, causing "overweight." But, above all, fats are the highest energy foods, with more calories per gram than any other foodstuff. When fats are eaten, one of three things can happen. The fats can be digested and burned immediately for energy. If there is an excess after digestion, it can be stored in the form of body fat. Finally, some fats may not be digested but are eliminated in the feces.

In addition to the above, which applies to fats (including oils) in general, there are certain dietary requirements called *essential fatty acids,* which are "essential for good health" in a manner very similar to vitamins. Indeed some writers on food call these vitamin F. The Food and Nutrition Board notes:

> The syndrome of essential-fatty-acid (EFA) deficiency as demonstrated in a variety of animal species includes dermatitis, impairment of growth and reproductive capacity, decreased efficiency of energy utilization, decreased resistance to certain stresses such as X-ray and ultraviolet light, and impairment of lipid [fat] transport.

Health writers discuss human cases of acne and eczema, swelling or edema, dry and brittle hair, loss of sex drive, a decline in the presence of desirable intestinal bacteria, dandruff, and other consequences of insufficient essential fatty acids.

There are only 3 of these EFA, bearing the names linoleic acid, linolenic acid, and arachidonic acid. These are often found mixed in vegetable oils. Good sources are corn, soybean, cottonseed, and peanut oils. Sunflower and safflower oils are even better sources. But olive oil has less EFA, and butter and coconut oil almost none.

There are actually two types of fats in the human diet, *saturated* and *unsaturated.* The difference is one of chemical structure. Saturated fats, it turns out, come mostly from animal foods. Included here is cholesterol, which now has a bad reputation because it is associated with arterial degeneration, heart disease, and strokes. But cholesterol is needed by the body; it is a necessary element in the manufacture of sex hormones, of vitamin D, and for other purposes. When there is insufficient cholesterol in the diet, the liver will manufacture it.

The other type of fat, primarily from vegetable and fish sources, is called unsaturated. Such fats are believed to be more beneficial, but the evidence is not complete. The American diet has seen a substantial change during the past twenty-five years in the type of fats eaten. Fewer and fewer saturated fats are now in the diet, and more and more unsaturated ones. But there is not much to show for the change. Heart and other related diseases seem to be continuing at the same or a faster rate.

The total amount of fat needed in the diet is another much-discussed matter. Because most Americans are overweight, it is felt that we are eating too much total fat. About 40 percent of our food calories, the units by which dietary energy is measured, come from fats and oils. Most authorities believe we would be a healthier and longer-lived people if this could be reduced to 25 to 30 percent.

The latest evidence seems to show that, except for overweight, it is not so much the presence of fats in the diet that is damaging as it is the *absence* of the vitamins needed to handle them. In certain experiments, animals were fed a high-saturated-fat diet and did get a fatty degeneration of their arteries and more heart attacks. But when vitamins and minerals were added, no such signs of circulatory disease occurred—the animals merely became obese. The B vitamins—especially choline, inositol, and niacin—and vitamin C may play a special protective role in the body's handling of saturated fats and oils.

In addition, unsaturated fats do increase the body's needs for vitamin E (which serves as an internal preservative, preventing these fats and oils from oxidizing or be-

coming rancid within the body). An increase in polyunsaturated oils or margarines, so heavily advertised today,
should call for a corresponding increase of vitamin E in the
diet.

For good health, then, we should all have some fats,
especially the needed amounts of the essential fatty acids,
but not too much. And we need the vitamins to metabolize
them properly.

Carbohydrates

Starches and *sugars* are the nutritive carbohydrate
energy foods; together they make up about 50 percent of
the food calories for the average American today. Over the
last fifty years the total carbohydrate intake has decreased
by almost 25 percent, as we now eat fewer cereal grains
and potatoes, but the consumption of sugars and syrups has
increased by about 25 percent, to the point where the average person eats about two pounds of refined white sugar
(sucrose) each week. As we know, much of this sugar may
be "hidden" in bakery goods, soft drinks, snacks, and the
like.

One result is widespread dental decay. Another may be a
mass decline in mental equanimity and performance, for,
as we shall see, this sugar is likely to start a complex bodily
reaction capable of producing irritability, mental foggi-
ness, unnecessary tension, and other disturbing symptoms.
Indeed, Dr. John Yudkin has informed us of British animal
experiments in which replacing starch in the diet (on
which the animals formerly thrived) by refined white sugar
led to extreme malnourishment, with attendant physical
signs and behavioral aberrations.

Ingested carbohydrates—both sugars and starches—are
mostly converted to the simple sugar *glucose* in the digestive tract, and this glucose then enters the bloodstream. A
proper blood glucose level is an absolute necessity for
human life. This level is regulated by the hormone insulin

(produced in the pancreas): more insulin, less blood glucose, and less insulin, more glucose. Diabetics are deficient in insulin production and their blood sugar level tends to rise, especially after they've eaten carbohydrates. Some of the excess sugar spills over into the urine as the body tries to protect the blood sugar level. Untreated, an overly high blood sugar level can lead to severe consequences, including coma and even death.

The reverse condition of low blood sugar, called *hypoglycemia*, is also damaging, causing fatigue, irritability, depression, hyperemotionalism, and also—in the extreme —coma and death. Certain parts of the body, particularly the brain and the retina of the eye, have a specific need for a constant supply of glucose. This is ordinarily furnished by the body's stores of carbohydrate, but when the insulin level is excessive, the blood sugar level can fall to a dangerously low level.

Paradoxically, in many people, this condition of high-insulin and low glucose is produced by *eating* sugar. Apparently the ingested sugar overstimulates the production of insulin, which then lowers the sugar content of the bloodstream. This is the condition called *reactive hypoglycemia*, that causes the midmorning slump after a breakfast of coffee and doughnuts, or afternoon fatigue following a luncheon with sweet desserts. All of the symptoms of low blood sugar arise from excessive sugar in the diet!

An official of the National Institutes of Health has told us privately that, in his opinion, as much as 87 *percent* of the adult population is suffering from this disorder, a result of our eating so much refined sugar. Certainly a general grouchiness and irritability seem a current and unwelcome aspect of American life. Despite obvious economic and social advances during past decades, every conceivable group seems to be on the march today, bitter and disgruntled, nasty and unfair, often carrying its grudges to extremes. Very little of a spirit of good-natured tolerance and compromise is in evidence.

Recent times have variously been labeled the Age of Conformity and the Age of Anxiety. Perhaps our own days could be called the Age of Irritability. Can it be, in fact, that just as cardiovascular diseases and cancer have become endemic, so also have irritability and grouchiness, owing to an acquired failing in the handling of excessive sugars in the diet?

Contributing to this condition is a lack of vitamins and minerals. Carbohydrate metabolism particularly requires the B vitamins and vitamin C. Refined white sugar enters the body in the form of "naked," or "empty," calories, without carrying along the vitamins and minerals to metabolize it. Thus it must draw on the body's reserves of these vitamins and acts as a vitamin drain. (The initial effects of a deficiency of several of these vitamins and minerals is also a decline in mental performance, a weakness of the mind similar to bodily weaknesses and similar to hypoglycemia.)

Thus vitamin supplements are all the more desirable when carbohydrates, especially sugar, are in the diet in excess.

Going the other way by avoiding all carbohydrates, a feature of several fad diets, is not to be recommended. A sudden cut-off of carbohydrates can be particularly dangerous because the body may respond by a derangement in the metabolism of fats, producing acidosis, a condition which can even be fatal. Dr. Neil Solomon notes that those who avoid all fruits, grains, starches, and sugars, and end up with low blood sugar, "complain of their mental efficiency being slowed down, dizziness, fatigue, extreme irritability, and in advanced cases, the possibility of loss of sight; indeed, even death can result ... people foolish enough to practice self-diagnosis and follow 'low-carbohydrate' fad diets may be headed for serious trouble."

For safety—and because the brain and eye particularly need glucose—a very low carbohydrate diet should always have the supervision of a physician. The simple and pleasant dietary practices we will later recommend to accompany the vitamin regimens can produce a proper weight loss, if needed, without this extreme step of avoiding all carbohydrates. Vitamins are not effective in a vacuum —they need other foodstuffs, including carbohydrates, to work their special powers.

Roughage

Do we really want to eat only concentrated, nutrition-packed foods?

Such is the diet of carnivorous animals, the meat-eaters with long sharp canine teeth and jaws that open and shut on a hinge. These are the animals whose exclusive food is the flesh of other animals, which is full of nutrition but which can also putrefy rapidly. The intestinal tracts of tigers, wolves, and other carnivores are generally short, averaging only *three* times the length of the body. Their food can be digested quickly, and the remains should be eliminated before they rot within the body.

These animals also have an acid saliva and an absence of active sweat glands over most of their body surface. Only their paws and noses usually perspire.

At the other end of the scale are the grass- and grain-eating animals—cattle, sheep, horses, and other herbivores. Their teeth are flat and their jaws move sideways for grinding. Their saliva is alkaline and they perspire over their entire bodies. Because their food requires a lengthy digestion, their intestinal canals average about *thirty* times the length of their bodies.

Somewhere in between is man. He and his closest mammalian neighbors, the apes and monkeys, share some of the anatomical and functional traits of both groups: teeth and jaws that are a compromise between the carnivore and herbivore types, alkaline saliva, active sweat glands over most of the body, and, above all, an intestinal tract that averages about *twelve* times the length of the body. In the natural state these traits are perfectly suited to a diet of fruits, nuts, berries, and some green vegetation. Meat can also be eaten, though this is a small part of the diet of man's primate relatives—insect grubs and similar small animals are eaten from time to time.

Above are some of the biological arguments that vegetarians have advanced to support their avoidance of meat. Millions of people certainly have lived long and nutritiously—and still do—on vegetable diets augmented by milk, dairy products, and eggs. (A pure vegetable diet is deficient or dangerously low in several human dietary necessities, particularly vitamin B12 but also riboflavin and other nutrients as well, unless great care is taken.)

Foods of plant origin do contain indigestible carbohydrate called *roughage*. Cellulose in leafy vegetables, wheat, and rice bran, and pectin in tree fruits, are examples. These add bulk to the diet. They fill out the intestinal tract, giving the muscles that surround it something to "grab," and so aid in moving the food along. This is why they are so often suggested in cases of bowel irregularity and constipation.

More important, population studies of societies that normally eat a high roughage diet have revealed interesting facts about several serious diseases. Appendicitis, peptic ulcer, diverticulitis (a painful inflammation of the large intestine that sends 200,000 Americans a year to the hospital) and cancer of the intestine and rectum are rare among such peoples. These illnesses do occur with greater frequency among Americans who eat much less roughage.

Cancer of the lower bowel, for example, is almost nonexistent among the high-roughage groups, who ordinarily pass stools three or four times daily. This type of cancer now ranks second among all cancer in the United States. It kills about 50,000 persons a year, about the same number as perish in automobile accidents. More roughage in the diet might be a valuable preventive against this mortal affliction.

A diet that is low in roughage does have its proper uses from time to time. A patient with an inflamed or infected intestinal tract is often placed temporarily on such a "low-residue" diet. The early astronauts whose space voyages lasted only a few days had no provisions for elimination. They ate a special low-residue diet and wore diaperlike garments during their short time aloft.

The peoples who have traditionally flourished on all-meat diets, such as the primitive Eskimo, have not restricted their food to the muscle meats. The organ meats and other soft tissues containing fiber, the marrow of bones, and even gnawed bones themselves, all added bulk to this diet.

Roughage, which we can obtain most easily from salads, unrefined wheat, rice and other grains, and fruits and vegetables, should also be part of every healthy adult diet.

CHAPTER 15

The "Official" Government Vitamin Quotas

What do you think might be a "minimal daily requirement" of the average person for *water?*

At first glance this question seems senseless, for we are all accustomed to drinking water or other liquids freely, more or less as our thirst dictates. Also, we know that the amount of water we need depends on several factors—how much salty food we have eaten, the temperature around us and the amount of perspiration we are prone to, our physical exertion, and so on. So the amount of water each of us needs does seem to be highly variable.

But a moment's reflection shows that under certain circumstances, the question still has to be answered. Those who prepare supplies for ships and submarines must estimate the amount of water needed by the "average" individual for drinking, as must those making up emergency rations for lifeboats and fallout shelters, and the diets of astronauts and others in isolated artificial environments.

But since the water needs will vary so much depending on the individual and the circumstances (including the remainder of the diet) any such estimate has to be a compromise. It will be based on assumptions of physical activity, total sweating, and diet that will be too low for some persons and too high for others. (Under the most favorable circumstances, by the way, which means absence of sweating, minimal physical activity, and a low-salt diet, the total water from all food and drink for an adult should be at least one and a half quarts per day.)

In a very similar way, the same variability, also affected by several types of causes, will influence the actual vitamin, mineral, and caloric needs of any particular individual on any given day. Tom is not the same biologically as Harry—and even if he were, his different meals and lifestyle would mean different nutrient needs. And Sally and Jane differ, too, both from Tom and Harry and from each other.

The Food and Nutrition Board's 1968 Recommended Daily Dietary Allowances

> The allowances are intended to serve as goals for planning food supplies and as guides for the interpretation of food consumption records of groups of people. The actual nutritional status of groups of healthy people or individuals must be judged on the basis of physical, biochemical, and clinical observations combined with observations of food or nutrient intakes.

So states the first page of *Recommended Dietary Allowances* (7th Revised Edition, 1968), published by the august Food and Nutrition Board. With proper scientific caution, the Board also admits that its recommendations have always been "value judgements based on the existing knowledge of nutritional science and were subject to revision as new knowledge became available."

In particular, the Board is careful to state clearly that its allowances for vitamins, minerals, and protein *"are not necessarily adequate to meet the additional requirements of persons depleted by disease, traumatic stresses, or prior dietary inadequacies."* (Emphasis added.)

In fact, its recommendations "should serve only as a reference . . . [because] In determining nutritional status, the current and past nutrient intake must be taken into consideration, as well as an evaluation of clinical signs and symptoms, growth and development, and biochemical data on tissue and excretory levels of nutrients."

The Food and Nutrition Board, a distinguished group of scientists and experts who serve without pay, was established as a part of the prestigious National Research Council of the National Academy of Sciences in 1940. Its first dietary "standards" were published in 1943, and they have been revised every several years since that time.

Shown here is the 1968 revision, which includes recommendations for 7 nutrients that had not been present in the previous 1963 version. These are the vitamins B_6, B_{12}, E, and folacin (folic acid), and the minerals phosphorus, iodine, and magnesium. Note that protein and calories (called "k-cal" on the chart) are included.

In addition to the nutrients on the chart, the Board also discusses other *essential* nutrients for which the listing of actual recommended dietary amounts is beyond the scope of present-day nutritional knowledge or is impossible because the requirements are affected by too many outside factors. These include (in the 1968 version) the vitamins biotin, choline, pantothenic acid, and vitamin K, and the minerals copper, fluorine, chromium, cobalt, manganese, molybdenum, selenium, zinc, sodium, potassium, and chloride.

What do the listings on the chart mean? Are they the actual amounts of vitamins, minerals, and protein that the average person needs each day?

To answer these questions, let us look at how these listings were arrived at. The Food and Nutrition Board made up two basic "typical" individuals, which they called the "reference man and woman." These were assumed to be 22 years old, living in a temperate climate, wearing proper clothing, and persons whose physical activity is "light"—that is, not too sedentary and not too arduous. The man was assumed to weigh 70 kilograms (kg) (154 lbs) and the woman 58 kg (128 lbs), and both of normal height. Most

FOOD AND NUTRITION BOARD, NATIONAI
RECOMMENDED DAILY
Designed for the maintenance of good nutrition

	AGE [b] (years) From Up to	WEIGHT (kg) (lbs)	HEIGHT cm (in.)	kcal	PROTEIN (gm)	FAT-SOLUBLE VITAMINS VITA-MIN A ACTIVITY (IU)	VITA-MIN D (IU)	VITA MIN ACTI (IU)
Infants	0 – 1/6	4 9	55 22	kg × 120	kg × 2.2 [c]	1,500	400	5
	1/6 – 1/2	7 15	63 25	kg × 110	kg × 2.0 [c]	1,500	400	5
	1/2 – 1	9 20	72 28	kg × 100	kg × 1.8 [c]	1,500	400	5
Children	1 – 2	12 26	81 32	1,100	25	2,000	400	10
	2 – 3	14 31	91 36	1,250	25	2,000	400	10
	3 – 4	16 35	100 39	1,400	30	2,500	400	10
	4 – 6	19 42	110 43	1,600	30	2,500	400	10
	6 – 8	23 51	121 48	2,000	35	3,500	400	15
	8 – 10	28 62	131 52	2,200	40	3,500	400	15
Males	10 – 12	35 77	140 55	2,500	45	4,500	400	20
	12 – 14	43 95	151 59	2,700	50	5,000	400	20
	14 – 18	59 130	170 67	3,000	60	5,000	400	25
	18 – 22	67 147	175 69	2,800	60	5,000	400	30
	22 – 35	70 154	175 69	2,800	65	5,000	—	30
	35 – 55	70 154	173 68	2,600	65	5,000	—	30
	55 – 75+	70 154	171 67	2,400	65	5,000	—	30
Females	10 – 12	35 77	142 56	2,250	50	4,500	400	20
	12 – 14	44 97	154 61	2,300	50	5,000	400	20
	14 – 16	52 114	157 62	2,400	55	5,000	400	25
	16 – 18	54 119	160 63	2,300	55	5,000	400	25
	18 – 22	58 128	163 64	2,000	55	5,000	400	25
	22 – 35	58 128	163 64	2,000	55	5,000	—	25
	35 – 55	58 128	160 63	1,850	55	5,000	—	25
	55 – 75+	58 128	157 62	1,700	55	5,000	—	25
Pregnancy				+200	65	6,000	400	30
Lactation				+1,000	75	8,000	400	30

[a] The allowance levels are intended to cover individual variations among most no: persons as they live in the United States under usual environmental stresses. The rec mended allowances can be attained with a variety of common foods, providing other nutri for which human requirements have been less well defined. See text for more-detailed dis sion of allowances and of nutrients not tabulated.

[b] Entries on lines for age range 22–35 years represent the reference man and woman at 22. All other entires represent allowances for the midpoint of the specified age range.

[c] The folacin allowances refer to dietary sources as determined by *Lactobacillus casei* as Pure forms of folacin may be effective in doses less than ¼ of the RDA.

CADEMY OF SCIENCES–NATIONAL RESEARCH COUNCIL
IETARY ALLOWANCES,ᵃ REVISED 1968
: practically all healthy people in the U.S.A.

| TER-SOLUBLE VITAMINS | | | | | | MINERALS | | | | |
FOLACIN[c†] (mg)	NIACIN (mg equiv)[d]	RIBOFLAVIN (mg)	THIAMIN (mg)	VITAMIN B_6 (mg)	VITAMIN B_{12} (μg)	CALCIUM (g)	PHOSPHORUS (g)	IODINE (μg)	IRON (mg)	MAGNESIUM (mg)
0.05	5	0.4	0.2	0.2	1.0	0.4	0.2	25	6	40
0.05	7	0.5	0.4	0.3	1.5	0.5	0.4	40	10	60
0.1	8	0.6	0.5	0.4	2.0	0.6	0.5	45	15	70
0.1	8	0.6	0.6	0.5	2.0	0.7	0.7	55	15	100
0.2	8	0.7	0.6	0.6	2.5	0.8	0.8	60	15	150
0.2	9	0.8	0.7	0.7	3	0.8	0.8	70	10	200
0.2	11	0.9	0.8	0.9	4	0.8	0.8	80	10	200
0.2	13	1.1	1.0	1.0	4	0.9	0.9	100	10	250
0.3	15	1.2	1.1	1.2	5	1.0	1.0	110	10	250
0.4	17	1.3	1.3	1.4	5	1.2	1.2	125	10	300
0.4	18	1.4	1.4	1.6	5	1.4	1.4	135	18	350
0.4	20	1.5	1.5	1.8	5	1.4	1.4	150	18	400
0.4	18	1.6	1.4	2.0	5	0.8	0.8	140	10	400
0.4	18	1.7	1.4	2.0	5	0.8	0.8	140	10	350
0.4	17	1.7	1.8	2.0	5	0.8	0.8	125	10	350
0.4	14	1.7	1.2	2.0	6	0.8	0.8	110	10	350
0.4	15	1.3	1.1	1.4	5	1.2	1.2	110	18	300
0.4	15	1.4	1.2	1.6	5	1.3	1.3	115	18	350
0.4	16	1.4	1.2	1.8	5	1.3	1.3	120	18	350
0.4	15	1.5	1.2	2.0	5	1.3	1.3	115	18	350
0.4	13	1.5	1.0	2.0	5	0.8	0.8	100	18	350
0.4	13	1.5	1.0	2.0	5	0.8	0.8	100	18	300
0.4	13	1.5	1.0	2.0	5	0.8	0.8	90	18	300
0.4	13	1.5	1.0	2.0	6	0.8	0.8	80	10	300
0.8	15	1.8	+0.1	2.5	8	+0.4	+0.4	125	18	450
0.5	20	2.0	+0.5	2.5	6	+0.5	+0.5	150	18	450

iacin equivalents include dietary sources of the vitamin itself plus 1 mg equivalent for 60 mg of dietary tryptophan.
ssumes protein equivalent to human milk. For proteins not 100 percent uitlized factors ld be increased proportionately.

scorbic Acid = Vitamin C
olacin = Folic Acid
ug = micrograms

important, both of these hypothetical reference people were assumed to be "normally healthy."

Exercising proper scientific caution, the Food and Nutrition Board has never claimed that most of us resemble the "typical" individuals on which their allowances are based. No one denies that the recommendations do not take into consideration the prior loss of nutrients in the processing, storage, cooking, or serving of food. Also, the allowances, based on short-term needs, are expected to cover good nutrition for the life span as a whole, though little is known of long-term requirements. The allowances admittedly apply only to persons in good health—the requirements of nutrients vary greatly under conditions of illness.

In her excellent work *The Science of Nutrition,* Professor Marian Thompson Arlin notes that these allowances are based on the "existing knowledge of nutritional science," and such knowledge "often consists of a few studies conducted on a handful of select individuals. Because healthy college students, particularly males, are often available as enthusiatic and cooperative research material (particularly when paid), the bulk of research tends to reflect the needs of this particular group, obviously not representative of the population as a whole."

She adds: *"Data that are available tend to delineate minimal rather than optimal needs"* (emphasis added), even though the allowances are intended to include a safety factor.

As an illustration of the cautious and reserved approach taken in preparing these allowances, glance at the table and note there are no vitamin D listings for adults over the age of twenty-two. The accompanying text, however, states clearly that "Vitamin D is essential at all ages for maintenance of calcium homeostasis [balance] and skeletal integrity." The omission of a specific vitamin D recommendation for adults thus does not mean that no vitamin D is needed, but that our nutritional knowledge is inadequate at present to specify a particular amount. The same is true for its 15 other nutrients mentioned as "essential," but not in the table.

How shall we interpret these recommendations? Professor Arlin notes that although they "were not designed to evaluate the adequacy of individual diets, they are frequently used for this purpose . . . *The most common error is failure to understand that they cannot be used to define the presence or absence of malnutrition.* This is because of the great individual variation in nutrient needs . . ." (Emphasis added.)

One suggested interpretation is that they can be used to assess the *risk* of malnutrition. That is, if the allowance for any one vitamin or mineral covers the needs of 95 percent of the normally healthy population, then 5 out of every 100 healthy people may have a greater need for it. The odds favor you, *if* you are normally healthy, falling into the 95 percent, but there is a 5 percent chance that your needs are greater. That is the risk you would take for this one particular vitamin or mineral if your intake were just to meet the recommended allowance.

But since there are many essential vitamins and minerals, and the individual variation is so great among different people, the chances are far, far higher than 5 percent that you would be in the "risk" category for at least one of these nutrients. The doctrine of "biochemical individuality" makes it very likely that each of us does need a much greater amount under *normal* conditions of one or another of these nutrients than is listed in the table.

Further, since stress and disease can increase our nutrient needs greatly, people whose health is not up to par often do demonstrably have their health improved by far greater amounts. Not all of us can hope to resemble in our own biology and chemistry the twenty-two-year-olds that served as a basis for these "Recommended Dietary Allowances" for adults.

The Food and Drug Administration's MDR's and U.S. RDA's

If the Food and Nutrition Board can make its recommendations from a detached and lofty scientific plane, the Food and Drug Administration has no such safe or sheltered position. It is out on the firing line, obligated by federal law to insure the safety and effectiveness of pharmaceutical and other drugs, and the purity and wholesomeness of our food. Often the FDA is caught in crossfires between various industry groups, consumer organizations, other government agencies, the press, medical groups, and so on.

The FDA got into the "vitamin business" in the 1960's. Of course, it has always been expected to protect the public from charlatans and deceitful merchants, so that, for example, the listed quantities of vitamins and minerals on a dietary supplement (vitamin pill or liquid) sold to the public should be as advertised. But in the 1960's the FDA went a good bit further.

It established vitamin "standards" and began to propose many limitations on admittedly nondangerous vitamin amounts. Many critics accused the FDA of using the vitamin issue as a smokescreen to avoid dealing with more serious matters, such as drug safety and the misleading packaging of foods. To investigate these other, more important issues would mean stepping on too many big business toes, said the critics, so the FDA used the vitamin issue (which it knew would attract much attention) to present the image of a vigorous regulating agency devoted to the public welfare.

This controversy continues to the present day, and we will discuss it later. At the moment, let us note that the earlier set of FDA vitamin standards were called Minimum Daily Requirements, abbreviated MDR's, and were supposed to be modeled after the Food and Nutrition Board's recommendations of the time (1963). But within the FDA there was a slip-up because somehow the amounts of the various vitamins got changed. The MDR's were substantially lower, when they were finally published, than the original recommendations.

Dr. William H. Sebrell, the chairman of the committee that had made the original recommendations for the National Research Council and the Food and Nutrition Board, denounced the FDA vitamin regulations. Even scientists within the FDA were opposed to them. The FDA commissioner, Dr. James Goddard at the time, went looking for the man who had changed the recommended amounts but found that he had left the agency. Dr. Goddard commented: "It shook me up that we didn't have enough know-how to prevent the mistakes that became apparent in the dietary supplement regulations."

But the bureaucracy could not change course and after they were published, by law, the MDR's became the standard listed on every vitamin label. Only 6 vitamins and 4 minerals were included, and some of these in amounts that were significantly lower than the scientific recommendations on which they were supposed to be based. For vitamin C, for example, the MDR for "adults" (twelve years or older) was only 30 mg, so vitamin pills containing this amount would in 1973 be labeled "100% Minimum Daily Requirement," or the equivalent, even though this is only half of the amount recommended in 1968 by the Food and Nutrition Board.

Public sentiment has caused tens of thousands of critical letters to be sent to the FDA about its approach to vitamin regulations. Congressmen and Senators have attacked it, as have newspaper columnists, both liberal and conservative. Most important, so have many scientists and food experts.

Without altering its basic approach, the FDA proposed a new set of regulatory vitamin standards in 1973. These are called the U.S. RDA, standing for U.S. Recommended *Daily* Allowances, and are listed in the following table. These are intended to be a shortened and simplified version of the 1968 Food and Nutrition Board's allowances in the previous table. Note that in addition to the nutrients listed, the FDA also recognizes the following vitamins and minerals as essential in human nutrition: vitamin K, choline, chlorine, potassium, sodium, sulfur, fluorine, and manganese. In the table below, "infant" means a baby under twelve months.

(The new regulations also propose controversial rules about vitamin labeling and the contents of vitamin and mineral pills and supplements, which matters we will discuss much later.)

Official Allowances for Animals

Interestingly, the nutritional recommendations of the National Research Council of the National Academy of Sciences are concerned with more than just human needs. The Food and Nutrition Board also makes recommendations for *animal* feeding through a Committee on Animal Nutrition. In 1962 this committee published *Nutrient Requirements for Laboratory Animals,* and thereby created a curious disparity, first pointed out by biochemist Irwin Stone in his 1972 book, *The Healing Factor: Vitamin C Against Disease.*

We know that most mammals produce the vitamin C they need within their own bodies, and that only man, his nearby ape and monkey primate neighbors, the guinea pig, and one species of bat, need vitamin C in their food. "The recommended diet for the monkey—our closest mammalian relative—is 55 milligrams of ascorbic acid per kilogram of body weight," Stone notes. "The daily amount suggested as adequate for the guinea pig varies depending upon which of two diets is selected and ranges from 42 mg to 167 mg per kilogram of body weight. . . ."

Thus a 70-kg (154 lb) monkey, if such could exist, would have a total recommended daily vitamin C intake of 3,850 mg (3.85 gm) and a hypothetical 70-kg (154 lb) guinea

U.S RECOMMENDED DAILY ALLOWANCE (U.S. RDA)
THE FOOD AND DRUG ADMINISTRATION, 1973

Vitamins & minerals[1]*	Unit of measurement	Infants	Children under 4 years of age	Adults and children 4 or more years of age	Pregnant or lactating women
Vitamin A	International units	1,500	2,500	5,000	8,000
Vitamin D	do	400	400	400	400
Vitamin E	do	5	10	30	30
Vitamin C	Milligrams	35	40	60	60
Folic acid	do	0.1	0.2	0.4	0.8
Thiamine	do	0.5	0.7	1.5	1.7
Riboflavin	do	0.6	0.8	1.7	2.0
Niacin	do	8	9	20	20
Vitamin B6	do	0.4	0.7	2.0	2.5
Vitamin B12	Micrograms	2	3	6	8
Biotin	Milligrams	0.15	0.15	0.30	0.30
Pantothenic acid	do	3	5	10	10
Calcium	Grams	0.6	0.8	1.0	1.3
Phosphorus	do	0.5	0.8	1.0	1.3
Iodine	Micrograms	45	70	150	150
Iron	Milligrams	15	10	18	18
Magnesium	do	70	200	400	450
Copper	do	0.6	1.0	2.0	2.0
Zinc	do	5	8	15	15

[1] The following synonyms may be added in parenthesis immediately following the name of the vitamin:

Vitamin	Synonym
Vitamin C	Ascorbic acid
Folic acid	Folacin
Riboflavin	Vitamin B2
Thiamine	Vitamin B1

* In addition to the vitamins and minerals listed . . ., vitamin K, choline, and the minerals chlorine, potassium, sodium, sulfur, fluorine, and manganese are recognized as essential in human nutrition, but no U.S. Recommended Daily Allowance (U.S. RDA) has been established for these nutrients.

(Federal Register, Volume 38, No. 148—Thursday, August 2, 1973) pig, a daily recommended intake between 2,940 and 11,690 mg (roughly 3 to 11½ gm). These figures suggest an interesting comparison. On an equivalent weight basis, an average 154-lb man would have a much higher vitamin C intake if he followed these *animal* guidelines rather than the guidelines for *human* nutrition set up by the Food and Nutrition Board. If you compare the average man to the hypothetical 154-lb monkey, the recommendation is 55 times the human guideline, and if you compare the guinea pig, it is 42 to 167 times the human guideline. Can our official nutritional agencies be shortchanging human needs in favor of animal needs?

It is interesting also that these higher amounts lie roughly within the 2 to 10 gm of daily intake that have been recommended by so many vitamin C proponents in recent years. These higher daily levels are so far above the amounts required to prevent obvious signs of scurvy (about 10 mg daily for the average adult human), or even the 60 mg of the U.S. RDA, that it is clear somebody is out of step. Scanning the dozens of medical references Irwin Stone cites, and reviewing personal experience with office patients, it seems evident that the U.S. RDA's are far from the optimal levels for the best health.

Albert Szent-Györgyi is one of the most honored and respected of modern chemists. Nobel Prize Laureate, MD and PhD, his prizewinning basic research dealt with human metabolism in general and ascorbic acid in particular. In 1972 he wrote, in a preface to Irwin Stone's book:

> I have always had the feeling that not enough use was made of it [vitamin C] in supporting human health. The reasons were rather complex. The medical profession itself took a very narrow and wrong view. Lack of ascorbic acid caused scurvy, so if there was no scurvy there was no lack of ascorbic acid. Nothing could be clearer than this. The only trouble was that scurvy is not a first symptom of lack but a final collapse, a premortal syndrome, and there is a very wide gap between scurvy and full health . . . Full

health, in my opinion, is the condition in which we feel best and show the greatest resistance to disease . . . If you do not have sufficient vitamins and get a cold, and as a sequence pneumonia, your diagnosis will not be "lack of ascorbic acid" but "pneumonia." So you are waylaid immediately. . . . Nor does wealth and rich food necessarily protect against lack of vitamins. I remember my contact with one of the wealthiest royal families of Europe where the young prince had constant temperature and had poor health. On administering vitamin C, the condition readily cleared up. . . .

For reasons such as these, many who have been engaged in the scientific study of nutrition have generally recommended doses of vitamins that are far above the "official" recommendations—and especially for persons subjected to the stresses of an over- or under-active existence, for those who do not eat consistently nutritious meals, or who cannot always be sure of the nutritional quality of the foods commonly available to them.

More Confusion

As if to mix things up even more, in 1974 the Food and Nutrition Board issued yet another set of "Recommended Dietary Allowances," just after the Food and Drug Administration had based its U.S. RDA's on the 1968 recommendations. These latest vitamin "quotas" are unfortunately mostly lower than previous standards.

Senator William Proxmire, Democrat of Wisconsin, has long been known as one legislator keenly interested in good health via nutrition and exercise. When the 1973 FDA vitamin and mineral rules were announced, he introduced a bill in the U.S. Senate (S. 2801) to overturn governmental restrictions on safe and harmless vitamin supplements. But when word reached him of the revision of the Food and Nutrition Board's latest Recommended Dietary Allowances, he made a biting speech in the Congress (June 10, 1974):

The Food and Drug Administration proposal to regulate safe vitamins and minerals as dangerous drugs if they exceed 150 percent of the so-called recommended daily allowance or recommended dietary allowance (RDA) of vitamins and minerals is based on an arbitrary, unscientific, and tainted standard. The RDA standard is established by the Food and Nutrition Board of the National Research Council, which is influenced, dominated, and financed in part by the food industry. It represents one of the most scandalous conflicts of interest in the Federal Government.

As author of a bill, S. 2801, which has 38 Senate cosponsors, which would prevent the FDA from putting its regulations into effect next January, I am particularly interested in this matter.

There are a dozen or more reasons why the so-called recommended daily allowance (RDA) is a capricious, unscientific, and illogical standard.

CONFLICTS OF INTEREST

First and foremost is the unconscionable conflict of interest of those on the Food and Nutrition Board which establishes it. The board is both the creature of the food industry and heavily financed by the food industry. It is the narrow economic interest of the industry to establish low official RDA's because the lower the RDA's the more nutritional their food products appear.

The board's industry liaison panels include breakfast food companies, candy makers, soft-drink producers, baking firms, and chemical corporations.

The present chairman of the Food and Nutrition Board, for example, occupies an academic chair funded by the Mead-Johnson baby food company. He appeared at the FDA vitamin hearings not only as an FDA-Government witness but also on behalf of such firms and groups as Mead-Johnson and Abbott Laboratories.

He was also scheduled to appear on behalf of the Pet Milk Co. and Distillation Products. His research was funded to the tune of about $40,000 by the FDA and he had additional Government grants of about $90,000 in the year he appeared for the FDA.

In the latest—1974—edition of the Food and Nutrition Board's recommended daily allowances, most values that were changed were lowered from previous standards. There is a very simple and quite unscientific reason for this.

With low RDA's the food companies which advise the Food and Nutrition Board can then print tables on their food packages making their products appear to contain a higher level of nutrients than if higher or optimum levels were established. When milk and fruit together provide as much nutritional value as the breakfast food they are eaten with, one can see how ridiculously low and self-serving the new low RDA standards really are.

VALUES FLUCTUATE CAPRICIOUSLY

A second reason why the RDA standards are suspect is that they have fluctuated capriciously from year to year both in the nutrients listed and in the recommended daily allowance. For example, in the recommendations by the board for pantothenic acid, a B complex vitamin, in the period 1964–74, it was not on the 1964 list, was listed at 5 milligrams on the next list, was not on the third list, was back at 5 milligrams on the fourth list, was doubled to 10 milligrams on the fifth list, and was removed completely from the latest 1974 edition.

Is it a drug? Is it not a drug? Under the proposed FDA regulations, 10 milligram capsules would have been regulated as a drug after the second and fourth editions of the RDA's, as a food or a food supplement under the fifth change, and ignored after the 1974 list.

In the 1968 RDA list, there were 55 changes in value from the 1964 list, varying from 20 to 700 percent. The latest—1974—list shows similar subjective and unscientific variations. In the 1964–74 period the RDA's recommended by the Food and Nutrition Board for a child of 4 have varied by 100 percent for vitamin A, 230 percent for vitamin E, 700 percent for folacin, 150 percent for vitamin

B–1, 122 percent for vitamin B–6, and 300 percent for vitamin B–12.

How can such an unstable standard be used to regulate vitamins? The RDA's are not scientific standards. They are little more than subjective, off-the-cuff and, in many cases, prejudiced values. . . .

. . . third, not only do the RDA's fluctuate capriciously and are established by those with overwhelming economic conflicts and self-serving interests, but there is a very considerable body of scientific evidence that the RDA's are ridiculously low. For example:

EXAMPLES OF LOW VALUES

Folacin. The RDA for folacin [folic acid] for some categories of individuals has varied by 700 percent in the last 10 years. It is now 400 micrograms for mature adults. The latest pronouncement cut the RDA for children in half. This has come at the very time the Canadian Government's nutritional survey found that half of all Canadians had "moderate deficiency" levels of folacin in their blood and that 10 percent of all Canadians were in the range of "high risk" deficiency.

There is strong evidence that the lack of folacin produces congenital deformities and increases the danger of accidental hemorrhage by fivefold. It is considered by some authorities as the most widespread deficiency in the United States, especially among pregnant women.

In light of such evidence, the RDA established for folacin by the Food and Nutrition Board appears to be dangerously low.

Vitamin B–6. The 1974 RDA for vitamin B–6 in 23–50-year-old females is 2 milligrams. But Dr. Paul Gyorgy, the eminent scientist who discovered vitamin B–6 recommended in 1971 that the general RDA for B–6 should be 25 milligrams a day or 12.5 times the present RDA. Women on the pill are especially subject to vitamin B–6 deficiency. Yet millions of women in the 23–50-year-old age group are told by the FDA and the Food and Nutrition Board that they can get a sufficient amount of B–6 at one-eighth the level which its discoverer recommends.

Vitamin C. There is now a very wide body of scientific evidence, in addition to the recommendation of Dr. Linus Pauling, the Nobel laureate, that the daily requirement for vitamin C is many times the 45 milligrams RDA now recommended by the Food and Nutrition Board. . . .

UNSCIENTIFIC STANDARD

The proposal to subject safe vitamins and minerals to regulation as drugs by the FDA if they are sold in quantities of 150 percent or more of the so-called RDA is a biased, unscientific, and capricious standard. At best the RDA's are only a "recommended" allowance at antediluvian levels designed to prevent some terrible disease. At worst they are based on the conflicts of interest and self-serving views of certain portions of the food industry. Almost never are they provided at levels to provide for optimum health and nutrition.

Our Own Vitamin Recommendations

In the next chapter we present the rejuvenative broad spectrum vitamin recommendations and regimens that are the main purpose of this book. These come from much library reading of the research of others, and certain theoretical considerations of our own. Most important, they come from *actual experience with human patients.*

It is a sad fact that many deriders of vitamin therapy, often nutritionists in high positions, are not physicians. They do not have the obligation of healing the sick or boosting health in living, breathing human beings on a daily basis. While they often scoff at vitamins, especially in hastily written newspaper and magazine articles, working physicians are finding many patients are strongly benefited by such nutritional enrichment, to the increase of the vitality and energy of their bodies and minds.

We do not know whether all the vitamin skeptics suffer the conflicts of interest and corruption described by Senator Proxmire or whether they are sincerely in error. We do know that good nutrition works to benefit health.

CHAPTER **16**:

A *Daily Vitamin* *Regimen for You*

The regimens below are for *adults* and are first arranged *by vitamin,* so we can explain the dosages of each, how to adjust these, and the necessary cautions. (We exclude children because of their rapid growth and greater biochemical individuality; vitamin regimens and dietary practices for children should be done on an individual basis by physicians well schooled in nutrition.) For each vitamin you will see categories by *age,* and then by *weight —underweight, normal weight,* and *overweight.* There are no hard-and-fast rules as to what "underweight" and "overweight" mean, because people vary in their muscle to fat ratio. But we ourselves know when we are excessively slender, with insufficient bodily mass for good health or whether we are overweight due to excess fat.

Examples:

Underweight	Male	5'7"	under 140 lbs
	Female	5'4"	under 105 lbs
Normal weight	Male	5'7"	150–160 lbs
	Female	5'4"	110–120 lbs
Overweight	Male	5'7"	over 175 lbs
	Female	5'4"	over 130 lbs

Those who are taller or shorter than these selected heights can readily judge for themselves whether their

193

body weight is too high or too low for their particular body frames.

Most vitamins are given in a *range* of desirable intake because of individual variability in body chemistry, life-style, dietary habits, exposure to stress, body frame, and so on. The *Explanation & Cautions* section for each vitamin should readily permit an excellent first approximation of a desirable starting intake.

Since each person's actual optimal vitamin needs will fluctuate on a day-to-day basis, just as the need for water or other food nutrients does, we cannot feel there is anything fixed or sacrosanct about the regimens below. They should be considered as guidelines, not as inflexible rules or per-manent formulas.

After one begins with a general program that approxi-mates a good level of vitamin supplementation, the levels should then be adjusted further, according to how one feels and responds. It is usually the case that you can trust your own bodily and mental feelings to know whether a particular dietary practice is good for you. A good health act is one that will produce feelings of well-being, whereas narcotics and addictive drugs (including alcohol) leave you feeling so bad later that there can be no doubt that they are harmful. Vitamins and other necessary nutrients in the proper amounts will do the opposite, leaving feelings of strength, vigor, and superior functioning.

After an arrangement by individual vitamins comes an arrangement of the same regimens by *age group*, so it will be easy to see the full array of suggested vitamin supple-ments for any individual. But be sure to read the *Explana-tion & Cautions* sections for each vitamin before attempt-ing to understand the total regimens.

Later we will have a special word for women, and notes as to the types of vitamins to take, and how to buy them. "All ages" in the following refers to those in the late teens and later years, not infants and children.

Remember, do not expect results the first few days. It often takes two weeks or longer before the desirable effects of vitamin supplementation manifest themselves.

Vitamin A

(in International Units)

Age Group		Male	Female
Late teens to 21		20,000–30,000	15,000–25,000
22 to 35	Underweight	20,000–30,000	15,000–25,000
	Normal weight	20,000	20,000
	Overweight	20,000	20,000
36 to 60	Underweight	20,000–30,000	15,000–20,000
	Normal weight	20,000	20,000
	Overweight	30,000	30,000
Over 60	Underweight	20,000–30,000	20,000–30,000
	Normal weight	20,000–30,000	20,000–30,000
	Overweight	20,000–30,000	20,000–30,000

EXPLANATION & CAUTIONS

More chemical stresses (air pollution, smoking, artificial additives in junky convenience foods, etc.), more vitamin A. Heavy use of the eyes for television viewing or under glaring lights, more vitamin A. Frequent eaters of salads, sweet potatoes, and liver should use the lower levels and can omit vitamin A supplements entirely if liver is eaten more than twice a week (one serving of calf or beef liver usually has about 50,000 IU's and chicken livers are roughly the same). Too much vitamin A can lead to falling hair, nausea, headaches—so if these occur, stop the supplements for a week to see if the vitamin A is the cause. (This is very unlikely at these low levels.) Inadequate vitamin A is a greater concern than overdosage and can bring about skin problems, increased infections, and even blindness. Older people with poor digestion should take the higher levels. Vitamin A is available in 10,000 IU capsules, so a

25,000 IU daily average can be achieved by taking two capsules one day and three the next, etc.

Vitamin D

(in International Units)

Age Group		Male	Female
Late teens to 21		800–1,200	800–1,200
	Underweight	400	400
22 to 35	Normal weight	800	800
	Overweight	800	800
	Underweight	400	400
36 to 60	Normal weight	800	800
	Overweight	800	800
	Underweight	800	800–1,200
Over 60	Normal weight	800	800–1,200
	Overweight	800	800–1,200

EXPLANATION & CAUTIONS

Vitamin D is a "growth" vitamin, with higher amounts required during childhood and the bone formation that continues into the late teens. Also, older persons, especially women, seem prone to bone weaknesses or absorption problems, so a higher intake should be desirable. Those who drink a quart of vitamin D-milk daily (which we do *not* recommend if the milk must be homogenized) are already receiving 400 IU's from this source, which can be taken into account. *Those who are frequently outdoors with many parts of the skin exposed to the sun can use the lower levels above or halve the indicated amounts.* Sunlight through glass (or smog-filled city air) loses its capacity to create vitamin D on the human skin. Vitamin D supplements are best taken along with calcium, especially in dolomite, a mineral supplement we will describe later. Overdoses of vitamin D are possible, so the quantities above should not be exceeded.

Vitamin E: Alpha-Tocopherol

(in International Units)

Age Group		Male	Female
Late teens to 21		200–800	200–600
22 to 35	Underweight	100–600	100–400
	Normal weight	200–600	200–400
	Overweight	400–800	400–600
36 to 60	Underweight	200–400	200–400
	Normal weight	400–1,200	400–1,200
	Overweight	600–1,200	600–1,200
Over 60	Underweight	600–800	600–800
	Normal weight	800–1,200	800–1,200
	Overweight	1,000–1,600	1,000–1,600

EXPLANATION & CAUTIONS

A more active life, more vitamin E. More exercise, more vitamin E. More polyunsaturated fats in the diet, more vitamin E. Higher weight and more body mass, also more vitamin E. *Women after menopause* have a heart attack rate that rises to come close to that of men—so also, more vitamin E. Older people can also benefit from higher vitamin E intake; notice how the lower levels go up in the table above with increasing age. Although the FDA states that vitamin E is "harmless," let us note again that *hypertensives (high blood pressure cases) and rheumatic heart disease sufferers should not begin high-level vitamin E regimens without medical supervision.* Many persons have undiagnosed high blood pressure, so if you are in doubt, take only 100–200 IU's until your blood pressure is checked.

Vitamin C: Abscorbic Acid

(in milligrams)

All ages and weights, male and female	1,000–5,000

EXPLANATION & CAUTIONS

We recommend beginning with 1,000 to 1,500 mg, depending on body size (large size, more vitamin). If one is prone to many colds and infections, 1,500–2,000 mg might be a more appropriate starting point. Smokers in particular can add an additional 500 milligrams at the start. More stress, more vitamin C. If a minor cold or allergy of the hay fever type seems to be coming on, increase the intake to 4,000–5,000 immediately. Later, if the symptoms seem to be disappearing, one can return to the lower levels. (In a later chapter we will describe in detail how the healthful preventive effects of such a vitamin C regimen was determined in a large-scale trial in 1972 with hundreds of subjects.) In rare cases of frequent colds, bleeding gums, many black-and-blue marks, etc., which persist despite such a regimen, higher daily intakes of 3,000 to 5,000 mg, even 5,000 to 10,000 mg (5 to 10 gm) may be attempted. Taking vitamin C (which is somewhat acid) after meals should eliminate any stomach distress, but if there is a slight bodily reaction, the *sodium ascorbate* form which has identical vitamin action can be taken. Only one caution attends vitamin C intake: *diabetics taking medicinal insulin should*

Vitamin B$_1$: Thiamin

(in milligrams)

Age Group		Male	Female
Late teens to 21		100–200	100–200
	Underweight	100–200	100–200
22 to 35	Normal weight	150–300	100–200
	Overweight	200–300	150–300
	Underweight	150–300	150–300
36 to 60	Normal weight	150–300	150–300
	Overweight	200–300	200–300
	Underweight	200–300	200–300
Over 60	Normal weight	200–300	200–300
	Overweight	200–300	200–300

have medical supervision when starting such a regimen (because vitamin C increases the efficiency of such insulin and can thus disrupt the sugar-insulin balance). All other persons can take even 10,000 mg daily or more without harm, and often with surprisingly beneficial results. The vitamin C intake should be spaced out evenly throughout the day, after meals and snacks.

EXPLANATION & CAUTIONS

Although thiamin is water soluble and harmless, there is still evidence that older persons use it less efficiently, hence the generally higher intakes suggested above with increasing age. Also, being a necessary part of all cellular metabolism, higher weights or larger body frames should lead to increased intake. Mental sluggishness, irritability, forgetfulness, etc., can all be results of lack of sufficient thiamin. But thiamin in such amounts should not be taken alone—all the B vitamins are needed together, so a high-level thiamin regimen alone is unlikely to be beneficial. Be sure to add the other B vitamins and vitamin C, when thiamin is taken.

Vitamin B₂: Riboflavin

(in milligrams)

Age Group		Male	Female
Late teens to 21		100–300	100–300
	Underweight	100–300	100–300
22 to 35	Normal weight	50–100	50–100
	Overweight	100–200	100–200
	Underweight	100–300	100–300
36 to 60	Normal weight	50–100	50–100
	Overweight	100–200	100–200
	Underweight	150–300	150–300
Over 60	Normal weight	150–300	150–300
	Overweight	150–300	150–300

EXPLANATION & CAUTIONS

Underweight persons who may be tense, withdrawn, anxious, depressed, etc., can benefit from higher riboflavin intakes, hence the higher starting levels in the underweight and younger age groups above. Recall the signs of riboflavin lack: cracks around the mouth and lips, purplish tongue, bloodshot eyes, a sensitivity to light. We are impressed with the animal experiments that demonstrate special cancer-inhibiting properties of riboflavin, and so recommend higher levels, as above, for older persons. In general, more tension and anxiety, more riboflavin. Heavier weight, larger body frame—more riboflavin. Less dairy products in the daily diet, also more riboflavin.

Vitamin B₃: Niacin

(in milligrams)

Age Group		Male	Female
Late teens to 21		200–2,000	200–2,000
	Underweight	400–2,000	400–2,000
22 to 35	Normal weight	200–1,000	200–1,000
	Overweight	300–1,000	300–1,000
	Underweight	300–2,000	300–2,000
36 to 60	Normal weight	200–1,000	200–1,000
	Overweight	300–1,000	300–1,000
	Underweight	400–2,000	400–2,000
Over 60	Normal weight	400–2,000	400–2,000
	Overweight	400–2,000	400–2,000

EXPLANATION & CAUTIONS

Recall the case of the Hong Kong Veterans and the history of pellagra. Later we will see that niacin has been the chief agent for the often-startling successes of "orthomolecular psychiatry," used to treat schizophrenia and autism. "Subclinical" pellagra, with symptoms of moodiness, disorientation, lack of ability to concentrate, anxiety, irritability, etc., may be widespread, and niacin has been successfully used to benefit many otherwise inexplicable cases of such distress, especially in younger people. (Since suicide is a leading cause of death among those in the Late Teens to 21 age group, 400 mg or more can be a suitable starting level in these ages, especially for tense and withdrawn "moody" individuals.) Tender gums, loss of appetite, headaches, depression—more niacin. Diarrhea and indigestion may also benefit from more niacin.

This vitamin comes in two chemical forms, *nicotinic acid* and *nicotinamide* (also called *niacinamide*). Recall that the former often causes a flushing or "tingling" in the extremities (especially the hands and forearms) within a few minutes after the vitamin is eaten. Some people enjoy this sensation because it tells them the vitamin is "working." This only lasts a few moments and tends to disappear after some weeks of high-level nicotinic acid intake. Nicotinamide does not have this effect, but there are reports from the Schizophrenia Foundation of New Jersey that nicotinamide has caused depression among some patients. *Therefore, we generally recommend the nicotinic acid form of niacin.* (Both forms of this vitamin are completely harmless.)

Vitamin B₆: Pyridoxine

(in milligrams)

Age Group		Male	Female
Late teens to 21		100–800	200–800
	Underweight	200–600	300–800
22 to 35	Normal weight	100–400	200–600
	Overweight	200–800	300–800
	Underweight	200–600	300–800
36 to 60	Normal weight	100–400	200–600
	Overweight	200–800	300–800
	Underweight	200–600	200–600
Over 60	Normal weight	100–400	100–600
	Overweight	300–800	300–800

Determine a starting level within the ranges indicated by gauging the efficiency of your own emotional and mental functionings—less efficiency, more niacin. Less alertness and cheerfulness, less feeling "at home" with reality, more niacin. More personal stress, more niacin. No other vitamin has been so effective in improving *the totality of consciousness* of many patients. The highest levels, in the 1,000-to-2,000-mg range, are only rarely needed and only for the most distressed. Again, niacin needs the other B vitamins and vitamin C to be most effective.

EXPLANATION & CAUTIONS

Dr. John M. Ellis has devised a simple Quick Early Warning (QEW) test for pyridoxine deficiency: extend your hand with palm up, wrist straight, and then attempt to bend the two joints in the four fingers (but not the knuckle joints in the hand itself) until the fingers reach the hand. (This is not the same as making a fist—only the two joints in each of the fingers is bent.) Do this with both hands. If there is any difficulty in having the finger joints bend and the tips cannot reach the hand, a pyridoxine deficiency is likely, and the higher-level dosages above are called for.

Vitamin B₁₂

(in micrograms)

Age Group		Male	Female
Late teens to 21		50–75	50–75
22 to 35	Underweight	25–75	50–100
	Normal weight	12–50	25–75
	Overweight	12–50	25–75
36 to 60	Underweight	25–75	50–100
	Normal weight	12–50	25–75
	Overweight	12–50	25–75
Over 60	Underweight	50–75	50–100
	Normal weight	25–75	25–75
	Overweight	25–75	25–75

Also, tense, worried, anxious persons can gain from more pyridoxine. Swellings of the feet, hands, around the cheekbones, and other signs of edema—more pyridoxine. *Pregnant and lactating women, women on the "pill," and those who have regular monthly menstrual edema (weight gain due to water retention) should take a minimal 300 mg daily.* More meat and fish—also more pyridoxine. No overdose is possible.

EXPLANATION & CAUTIONS

Exactly the reverse of pyridoxine, higher levels of vitamin B_{12} are desirable when *less* meat, fish, or dairy products are eaten. *Vegetarians should thus take higher amounts, within the indicated ranges.* Women in the child-bearing ages (that is, menstruating, pregnant, or lactating women) may also need more vitamin B_{12}, this vitamin being so important for the proper formation of the blood. Irregular menses, also more vitamin B_{12}. Those who are frail, underweight, "anemic," or physically weak may benefit from additional vitamin B_{12}, so higher levels are indicated for the "Underweight" in the table above. For inexplicable fatigue, more vitamin B_{12}. Also, older persons should be especially sure to maintain an adequate vitamin B_{12} intake (the Food and Nutrition Board notes special absorption difficulties for this vitamin with advanced age), especially since the elderly are more prone to pernicious anemia. No "cautions" are needed for vitamin B_{12}; it is safe in all amounts. Remember that this vitamin is measured in *micrograms*.

B Vitamin—Biotin

(in milligrams)

All ages and weights, male and female   0.3–0.6

EXPLANATION & CAUTIONS

Biotin is generally ignored because deficiencies are so rare, but the skin rashes, scaliness, hair loss, Leiner's disease (red skin) known to be caused by a lack of biotin, plus other unknown effects, have led us to include this vitamin in our regimens. More research needs to be done, but the general benefits with office patients of broad-spectrum vitamin regimens including biotin have been so pronounced that if possible (and on the general principle that B vitamins work best together) biotin should be included. *If possible?* We make this qualification because separate biotin supplements are hard to find. Manufacturers are behind on their ability to manufacture this vitamin, and most that is produced commercially goes into "multivitamin" tablets or capsules. The new FDA regulations will make biotin only an "optional" ingredient of multivitamin supplements, so careful label reading will be required to be sure that one does get supplements containing biotin. This essential vitamin is perfectly safe, so intakes of two or three or more times the amount above should not be feared, and may even be beneficial.

B Vitamin—Choline

(in milligrams)

All ages and weights, male and female   250–1,000

EXPLANATION & CAUTIONS

Younger people, except the overweight, should begin with 250 mg of choline daily. For the overweight, 500 mg may be a more suitable starting amount. More fats and carbohydrates in the diet—more choline. Men in the mature years after thirty-five should also, we feel, move up to 500 mg of choline, and women should make this increase after menopause, when they become more heart attack prone. Older persons, especially the overweight, may be benefited more by intakes in the 750-to-1,000-mg range. Choline is most important for many circulatory afflictions (arteriosclerosis, heart attacks, strokes, and related kidney disorders), so "high risk" individuals—smokers, the overweight, persons with a family history of such disorders —have a greater reason for adequate choline intake. (We will later describe some of the clinical work with heart attack recovery patients that leads to these conclusions.) The normally healthy individual can benefit from a reduction in cholesterol and triglycerides in the bloodstream that choline can produce, with a resultant gain in physical vigor and mental acuity. No choline "overdose" is possible. (Unfortunately, and inexplicably, choline is omitted from the permissible vitamins in multivitamin supplements by the new proposed FDA regulations—despite its recognition as "essential" by the Food and Nutrition Board of the National Research Council, National Academy of Sciences.)

B Vitamin—Folic Acid

(in milligrams)

All ages and weights, male and female   2–5

EXPLANATION & CAUTIONS

The newest investigations and theory published by Dr. Kurt A. Oster in November, 1973, is causing us to revise our thinking about folic acid. Office patients have been receiving supplements in the 0.1 to 1 mg range, as part of a general vitalizing B complex regimen. Now it appears that gout-prone and atherosclerotic (especially elderly diabetics) patients under medical care can be aided by 40–80 mg daily therapeutic intake—we will describe this surprising clinical work later. For "normally healthy" adults we now recommend intake in the 2-to-5-mg range. Men can begin with 2 to 3 mg, but women before menopause should take 3 to 5 mg, because folic acid is also important for the manufacture and growth of red blood cells. Fewer green vegetables (spinach, dark green lettuce, etc.) in the diet, more folic acid. Irregular or excessive menses, more folic acid. *Older persons of both sexes over sixty should have intake in the 4-to-5-mg range* because this vitamin may improve circulation, reduce the chances of gout (and related gouty arthritis and other complaints), and help repair damaged arteries. The new FDA regulations will permit nonprescription supplements containing 0.4 mg in tablets or capsules for ordinary adults, and 0.8 mg in supplements labeled "for pregnant or lactating women." Three to six capsules of the latter daily will meet this desirable range of folic acid intake.

B Vitamin—Inositol

(in milligrams)

Age Group		Male	Female
Late teens to 21		500	500
	Underweight	500	500
22 to 35	Normal weight	500	500
	Overweight	750–1,000	750–1,000
	Underweight	500	500
36 to 60	Normal weight	750–1,000	500–1,000
	Overweight	750–1,000	750–1,000
	Underweight	1,000	1,000
Over 60	Normal weight	1,000	1,000
	Overweight	1,000	1,000

EXPLANATION & CAUTIONS

This vitamin is a partner to choline; both work together to form lecithin, which is a fatlike substance that, instead of being deposited on arterial and other blood vessel walls, circulates in the bloodstream and may dissolve such deposits. Many of the remarks about choline apply to inositol: it is also harmless, believed to be especially beneficial to those in the "high risk" category for circulatory diseases, etc. Women after menopause should increase their inositol intake to equal that of men, and older persons have a greater need for blood vessel integrity and more inositol. Some cases of baldness have been cited as aided by inositol—attributed to improved circulation in the scalp— but no office patients have experienced this miracle, and we must view the claim with skepticism. More fats in the diet, more inositol. Smoking, more inositol. Air pollution, more inositol.

B Vitamin—PABA (Para-aminobenzoic Acid)

(in milligrams)

Age Group		Male	Female
Late teens to 21		50–100	50–100
	Underweight	100	100
22 to 35	Normal weight	100	100
	Overweight	100–200	100 200
	Underweight	100	100
36 to 60	Normal weight	100	100
	Overweight	100–200	100–200
	Underweight	200	200
Over 60	Normal weight	200	200
	Overweight	200–400	200–400

EXPLANATION & CAUTIONS

Higher body weights and larger body frames, more PABA. Increasing age, as shown, also more PABA. This vitamin may be antiarthritic and should be a part of a broad-spectrum B vitamin regimen. No personal office patients have had color restored to graying hair by PABA, but reports also persist that this has occurred. There are no cautions for PABA, which is harmless at all levels of intake.

B Vitamin—Pantothenic Acid

(in milligrams)

Age Group		Male	Female
Late teens to 21		50–100	50–100
	Underweight	100–200	100–200
22 to 35	Normal weight	100–200	100–200
	Overweight	100–300	100–300
	Underweight	100–200	100–200
36 to 60	Normal weight	100–200	100–200
	Overweight	100–300	100–300
	Underweight	100–200	100–200
Over 60	Normal weight	100–200	100–200
	Overweight	100–300	100–300

EXPLANATION & CAUTIONS

Pantothenic acid is a known antistress agent, so more stress (fatigue, anxiety, infection, etc.), more pantothenic acid. More body weight, also more vitamin. This vitamin works with vitamin C and cholesterol to produce important hormones in the adrenal cortex, but little is known of the body's optimal intake, so the regimens above are intended to provide a margin of safety. Pantothenic acid is an important constituent of "royal jelly," the substance that keeps honey bee larvae from turning into sterile, short-lived worker bees and, instead, permits them to develop into exceedingly fertile queen bees with great longevity. This is some indication of its metabolic power.

Pantothenic acid is easily destroyed in food processing and cooking, and may be especially important to those threatened by arthritis. Arthritis itself (or a family history thereof)—more pantothenic acid! Longevity experiments with animals (to be described later) indicate many possible benefits from a high-level pantothenic acid regimen. *Calcium pantothenate* is an alternative and usable chemical form of the vitamin. Both forms of the vitamin are harmless.

EFA—Essential Fatty Acids

(in grams)

Age Group		Male	Female
Late teens to 21		10–20	10–20
	Underweight	20–30	20–30
22 to 35	Normal weight	10–20	10–20
	Overweight	10–20	10–20
	Underweight	20–30	20–30
36 to 60	Normal weight	10–20	10–20
	Overweight	10–20	10–20
	Underweight	20–30	20–30
Over 60	Normal weight	10–20	10–20
	Overweight	10–20	10–20

EXPLANATION & CAUTIONS

Strictly speaking, the Essential Fatty Acids are not vitamins because they are required in *gram,* rather than milligram or smaller amounts, for good health. We include them here because of their importance to general vitality, sex drive, proper water balance, absorption of vitamins, clear skin, and healthy hair, etc. But the EFA are not purchased in pill form, neither tablets nor capsules. They are best obtained from oils (sunflower, safflower, corn, cottonseed, soybean, peanut oil—but not olive oil) used in salad dressings or for cooking. (Normal frying does not alter these important, essential fats.) One tablespoon or two of such oils as a total daily intake will meet the general needs of adults; underweight people may benefit from a bit more. Remember that *cold-pressed* and *expeller-pressed* oils are preferable, though ordinary vegetable oils have these EFA, too.

Vitamin Regimens at a Glance

On the following pages, the vitamin regimens are rearranged by *age group,* so one can see at a glance the total array of desirable vitamin supplementation (except that vitamin P, together with mineral supplements and other beneficial dietary practices, will be discussed in a later chapter). But look back at the preceding pages to be able to tailor a full regimen to the needs of any particular individual—that is, to gauge a good starting level for each vitamin within the indicated ranges.

We will also make some comments about the common characteristics of the various ages of life, as related to the totality of problems and habits that face all of us—the common biomedical experiences of humanity, so to speak.

The Last Years of True Physical Growth: 17 to 21

For most people, the body continues to develop both its hard and soft tissues—bones, muscles, and other parts —until the late teens or early twenties. After about 21 or 22, any further weight gain is likely to be fat, except for muscular growth that comes from a conscious exercise program.

During these last of the growing years, vitamin D and calcium are still necessary for bone development. Protein (and the vitamins and minerals to metabolize it) needs are above the demands of tissue regeneration, for the body frame is often still being filled out. These years can be physically energetic and more athletic teenagers may need the larger amounts of vitamin E.

Suicide due to depression ranks as the second or third cause of death during these years, so the vitamins that help reduce the mental effects of personal stress, and are especially useful with anxious, nervous, or withdrawn personalities, can be most significant: *Vitamin C* and the B vitamins *riboflavin, pantothenic acid, pyridoxine,* and above all, *niacin* (in the *nicotinic acid* form).

Late Teens to 21

	Male	Female	Units
Vitamin A	20,000–30,000	15,000–25,000	IU
Vitamin D	800–1,200	800–1,200	IU
Vitamin E	200–800	200–600	IU
Vitamin C (Ascorbic Acid)	1,000–5,000	1,000–5,000	mg
The B Vitamins			
Vitamin B_1 (Thiamin)	100–200	100–200	mg
Vitamin B_2 (Riboflavin)	100–300	100–300	mg
Vitamin B_3 (Niacin)	200–2,000	200–2,000	mg
Vitamin B_6 (Pyridoxine)	100–800	200–800	mg
Vitamin B_{12}	50–75	50–75	mcg
Biotin	0.3–0.6	0.3–0.6	mg
Choline	250–1,000	250–1,000	mg
Folic Acid	2–5	2–5	mg
Inositol	500	500	mg
PABA			
(Para-aminobenzoic Acid)	50–100	50–100	mg
Pantothenic Acid	50–100	50–100	mg
EFA			
(Essential Fatty Acids)	10–20	10–20	gm

Young Adulthood: 22 to 35

These are the years of peak physical strength, as a glance at the roster of any professional athletic team will show instantly. They are also the years when many of life's important patterns are established: the solidification of habits of marriage, child-rearing, behavior at work and in social life—and also, important habits of food, drink, and physical exercise.

Tendencies to obesity, alcoholism, nervousness, or other forms of physical or mental damage tend to become manifest during this period, as the actual obligations of adult life become evident.

Young manhood and young womanhood now begin

many of life's major challenges, including those to their health. Will this be a time when a sedentary existence becomes fixed, or will patterns of healthy exercise be started? Will excesses in food and alcoholic drink destroy health at a rapid pace, or will moderate and balanced practices lead to continued vigor and achievement?

Mental illness is not infrequent at this time, so special

Ages 22 to 35: Underweight

	Male	Female	Units
Vitamin A	20,000–30,000	15,000–25,000	IU
Vitamin D	400	400	IU
Vitamin E	100–600	100–400	IU
Vitamin C (Ascorbic Acid)	1,000–5,000	1,000–5,000	mg
The B Vitamins			
Vitamin B$_1$ (Thiamin)	100–200	100–200	mg
Vitamin B$_2$ (Riboflavin)	100–300	100–300	mg
Vitamin B$_3$ (Niacin)	400–2,000	400–2,000	mg
Vitamin B$_6$ (Pyridoxine)	200–600	300–800	mg
Vitamin B$_{12}$	25–75	50–100	mcg
Biotin	0.3–0.6	0.3–0.6	mg
Choline	250–1,000	250–1,000	mg
Folic Acid	2–5	2–5	mg
Inositol	500	500	mg
PABA (Para-aminobenzoic Acid)	100	100	mg
Pantothenic Acid	100–200	100–200	mg
EFA (Essential Fatty Acids)	20–30	20–30	gm

Ages 22 to 35: Normal Weight

	Male	Female	Units
Vitamin A	20,000	20,000	IU
Vitamin D	800	800	IU
Vitamin E	200–600	200–400	IU
Vitamin C (Ascorbic Acid)	1,000–5,000	1,000–5,000	mg

The B Vitamins

	Male	Female	Units
Vitamin B₁ (Thiamin)	150–300	100–200	mg
Vitamin B₂ (Riboflavin)	50–100	50–100	mg
Vitamin B₃ (Niacin)	200–1,000	200–1,000	mg
Vitamin B₆ (Pyridoxine)	100–400	200–600	mg
Vitamin B₁₂	12–50	25–75	mcg
Biotin	0.3–0.6	0.3–0.6	mg
Choline	250–1,000	250–1,000	mg
Folic Acid	2–5	2–5	mg
Inositol	500	500	mg
PABA (Para-aminobenzoic Acid)	100	100	mg
Pantothenic Acid	100–200	100–200	mg

EFA (Essential Fatty Acids)   10–20   10–20   gm

Ages 22 to 35: Overweight

	Male	Female	Units
Vitamin A	20,000	20,000	IU
Vitamin D	800	800	IU
Vitamin E	400–800	400–600	IU
Vitamin C (Ascorbic Acid)	1,000–5,000	1,000–5,000	mg

The B Vitamins

	Male	Female	Units
Vitamin B₁ (Thiamin)	200–300	150–300	mg
Vitamin B₂ (Riboflavin)	100–200	100–200	mg
Vitamin B₃ (Niacin)	300–1,000	300–1,000	mg
Vitamin B₆ (Pyridoxine)	200–800	300–800	mg
Vitamin B₁₂	12–50	25–75	mcg
Biotin	0.3–0.6	0.3–0.6	mg
Choline	250–1,000	250–1,000	mg
Folic Acid	2–5	2–5	mg
Inositol	750–1,000	750–1,000	mg
PABA (Para-aminobenzoic Acid)	100–200	100–200	mg
Pantothenic Acid	100–300	100–300	mg

EFA (Essential Fatty Acids)   10–20   10–20   gm

attention should be paid to the antistress vitamins—in particular, if one is "nervous," or high-strung. As before, an athletic life calls for the higher levels of vitamin E.

Women seeking to preserve their beauty should keep their total nutrition up to par. Graying hair may call for attention to PABA and pantothenic acid, skin and hair problems for attention to vitamin A and the EFA. But all the vitamins are important, so a complete program offers the best chances for the healthful look, which increasingly becomes the beautiful one as time passes during these years.

The Years of Maturity: 36 to 60

Physical growth is over (or should be), the patterns of life have usually established themselves, and the wisdom of experience leads for most to life's major accomplishments and achievements during this period.

Care must be taken that neither success nor failure at any given time leads to dietary indiscretions or excessive use of alcohol or drugs. The body's recuperative powers, while still present, are no longer as strong or responsive as they were at earlier ages. The common tragedies of life—the death of parents and other loved ones, business or career failures, marital discords or separations, and others—must not be allowed to affect one's health or health practices.

Paradoxically, career success as well as failure has often led to self-destruction or breakdown. Strength and vigor can be maintained during this period by proper diet and exercise—or, without these, there will be a progressive weakening of both body and mind.

Women face the special problems of *menopause* during this time, all of which will be accentuated and made more troublesome unless extra care is taken in dietary matters. The sex hormones are closely related to vitamins and minerals, and proper dietary supplements may make hormonal treatment more effective or even unnecessary.

This is the quarter century when the problems of youth have gone. Understanding and knowledge of life can make these years the most fulfilling of all when good health is present.

Ages 36 to 60: Underweight

	Male	Female	Units
Vitamin A	20,000–30,000	15,000–20,000	IU
Vitamin D	400	400	IU
Vitamin E	200–400	200–400	IU
Vitamin C (Ascorbic Acid)	1,000–5,000	1,000–5,000	mg

The B Vitamins

	Male	Female	Units
Vitamin B1 (Thiamin)	150–300	150–300	mg
Vitamin B2 (Riboflavin)	100–300	100–300	mg
Vitamin B3 (Niacin)	300–2,000	300–2,000	mg
Vitamin B6 (Pyridoxine)	200–600	300–800	mg
Vitamin B12	25–75	50–100	mcg
Biotin	0.3–0.6	0.3–0.6	mg
Choline	250–1,000	250–1,000	mg
Folic Acid	2–5	2–5	mg
Inositol	500	500	mg
PABA (Para-aminobenzoic Acid)	100	100	mg
Pantothenic Acid	100–200	100–200	mg

EFA (Essential Fatty Acids)	20–30	20–30	gm

Ages 36 to 60: Normal Weight

	Male	Female	Units
Vitamin A	20,000	20,000	IU
Vitamin D	800	800	IU
Vitamin E	400–1,200	400–1,200	IU
Vitamin C (Ascorbic Acid)	1,000–5,000	1,000–5,000	mg

The B Vitamins

Vitamin B1 (Thiamin)	150–300	150–300	mg
Vitamin B2 (Riboflavin)	50–100	50–100	mg
Vitamin B3 (Niacin)	200–1,000	200–1,000	mg
Vitamin B6 (Pyridoxine)	100–400	200–600	mg
Vitamin B12	12–50	25–75	mcg
Biotin	0.3–0.6	0.3–0.6	mg
Choline	250–1,000	250–1,000	mg
Folic Acid	2–5	2–5	mg
Inositol	750–1,000	500–1,000	mg
PABA			
(Para-aminobenzoic Acid)	100	100	mg
Pantothenic Acid	100–200	100–200	mg

EFA			
(Essential Fatty Acids)	10–20	10–20	gm

Ages 36 to 60: Overweight

	Male	Female	Units
Vitamin A	30,000	30,000	IU
Vitamin D	800	800	IU
Vitamin E	600–1,200	600–1,200	IU
Vitamin C (Ascorbic Acid)	1,000–5,000	1,000–5,000	mg

The B Vitamins

Vitamin B1 (Thiamin)	200–300	200–300	mg
Vitamin B2 (Riboflavin)	100–200	100–200	mg
Vitamin B3 (Niacin)	300–1,000	300–1,000	mg
Vitamin B6 (Pyridoxine)	200–800	300–800	mg
Vitamin B12	12–50	25–75	mcg
Biotin	0.3–0.6	0.3–0.6	mg
Choline	250–1,000	250–1,000	mg
Folic Acid	2–5	2–5	mg
Inositol	750–1,000	750–1,000	mg
PABA			
(Para-aminobenzoic Acid)	100–200	100–200	mg
Pantothenic Acid	100–300	100–300	mg

EFA			
(Essential Fatty Acids)	10–20	10–20	gm

The Golden Older Years: Over 60

Now we know that health and vigor need not precipitously decline when one is over 60. A full quarter of a century or more of vitality, strength, mental efficiency, and sexual interest and performance can be the return to those who have—and continue—good health practices.

Why do older people have special vitamin and mineral needs? There are several reasons:

- *Malabsorption.* Weaknesses in the digestive enzymes often lead to a lowered absorption of needed nutrients into the body. Sometimes supplementation of these enzymes is a part of the medical treatment of older people, but increased nutrients themselves in the diet will help by providing a greater chance of absorption. This is especially true for many minerals and the fat-soluble vitamins.

- A *lessening of physical activity* leads to a lowered need for caloric food energy and usually to a lessened total food intake. Also, *a decline in taste sensation* often leads to a smaller amount of food eaten. The less food eaten, the less vitamins and minerals ingested with these foods. Reducing a normal amount of foodstuffs by one-third, for example, will reduce the vitamins and minerals entering the body by the same amount, unless there is additional supplementation.

- *Dental problems* may give rise to a change in the diet. Less fresh fruit and vegetables may be eaten by those who cannot chew well. This also reduces the total amount of vitamins and minerals that are taken in, without additional supplementation.

- *Loneliness* is a frequent condition of old age. People who are alone often forgo the trouble of preparing nourishing meals. They nibble and snack, frequently on easily prepared foods (toast and margarine or jelly, tea, etc.) that are not nutritious.

• *Lowered incomes* lead to less funds available for food purchases among many older people. The cheaper, less nutritious foods may predominate in the diet, leading to vitamin and mineral deficiencies.

• A *lifetime accumulation* of deleterious substances (pesticides and other poisons, for example) and radiation (including natural radiation from the sun, cosmic rays, earth components, as well as from man-made fallout) can all weaken the body tissues and increase their need for the restorative effects of vitamins.

• *Illness and chronic complaints* can be accentuated in the aged owing to a lifetime of bad dietary habits, smoking, alcoholic intake, fatty degeneration of the arteries, and so on. Thus the starting point toward health is further back, so to speak. The body's resources may be continually depleted in combating such illnesses.

• *On the cellular level,* aging means "older" enzymes, which are less efficient. In a later chapter we will discuss this finding of "molecular biology," the newest branch of biological science, which may have discovered a most important clue to the very process of aging itself. As we will see, an *abundance* of vitamins around each cell can partially overcome the chemical effects of this inevitable process. This may help explain both the fact that older persons tend to use some water-soluble vitamins (which are always well-absorbed) "less efficiently," as the Food and Nutrition Board notes, and also the fact that older persons often do report substantially increased feelings of well-being and vitality from extra-large vitamin dosages.

Thus, though the total body size may decline in older persons, their vitamin and mineral needs do not go down at the same time.

Easily broken bones that will not heal, impaired vision, forgetfulness, loss of ability to concentrate, skin rashes, dental weaknesses, inexplicable bumps and bruises, various swellings, varicose veins, "burning soles," leg and other cramps, heart palpitations, and many other medical conditions have now been found often to respond to therapeutic vitamin and mineral dosages. One noted psychiatrist maintains that senility itself may be just a form of chronic malnutrition.

Ages Over 60: Underweight

	Male	Female	Units
Vitamin A	20,000–30,000	20,000–30,000	IU
Vitamin D	800	800–1,200	IU
Vitamin E	600–800	600–800	IU
Vitamin C (Ascorbic Acid)	1,000–5,000	1,000–5,000	mg

The B Vitamins

	Male	Female	Units
Vitamin B₁ (Thiamin)	200–300	200–300	mg
Vitamin B₂ (Riboflavin)	150–300	150–300	mg
Vitamin B₃ (Niacin)	400–2,000	400–2,000	mg
Vitamin B₆ (Pyridoxine)	200–600	200–600	mg
Vitamin B₁₂	50–75	50–100	mcg
Biotin	0.3–0.6	0.3–0.6	mg
Choline	250–1,000	250–1,000	mg
Folic Acid	2–5	2–5	mg
Inositol	1,000	1,000	mg
PABA			
(Para-aminobenzoic Acid)	200	200	mg
Pantothenic Acid	100–200	100–200	mg

EFA

	Male	Female	Units
(Essential Fatty Acids)	20–30	20–30	gm

Ages Over 60: Normal Weight

	Male	Female	Units
Vitamin A	20,000–30,000	20,000–30,000	IU
Vitamin D	800	800–1,200	IU
Vitamin E	800–1,200	800–1,200	IU
Vitamin C (Ascorbic Acid)	1,000–5,000	1,000–5,000	mg

The B Vitamins

Vitamin B₁ (Thiamin)	200–300	200–300	mg
Vitamin B₂ (Riboflavin)	150–300	150–300	mg
Vitamin B₃ (Niacin)	400–2,000	400–2,000	mg
Vitamin B₆ (Pyridoxine)	100–400	100–600	mg
Vitamin B₁₂	25–75	25–75	mcg
Biotin	0.3–0.6	0.3–0.6	mg
Choline	250–1,000	250–1,000	mg
Folic Acid	2–5	2–5	mg
Inositol	1,000	1,000	mg
PABA			
(Para-aminobenzoic Acid)	200	200	mg
Pantothenic Acid	100–200	100–200	mg

EFA			
(Essential Fatty Acids)	10–20	10–20	gm

Ages Over 60: Overweight

	Male	Female	Units
Vitamin A	20,000–30,000	20,000–30,000	IU
Vitamin D	800	800–1,200	IU
Vitamin E	1,000–1,600	1,000–1,600	IU
Vitamin C (Ascorbic Acid)	1,000–5,000	1,000–5,000	mg

The B Vitamins

Vitamin B₁ (Thiamin)	200–300	200–300	mg
Vitamin B₂ (Riboflavin)	150–300	150–300	mg
Vitamin B₃ (Niacin)	400–2,000	400–2,000	mg
Vitamin B₆ (Pyridoxine)	300–800	300–800	mg
Vitamin B₁₂	25–75	25–75	mcg
Biotin	0.3–0.6	0.3–0.6	mg
Choline	250–1,000	250–1,000	mg
Folic Acid	2–5	2–5	mg
Inositol	1,000	1,000	mg
PABA			
(Para-aminobenzoic Acid)	200–400	200–400	mg
Pantothenic Acid	100–300	100–300	mg

EFA			
(Essential Fatty Acids)	10–20	10–20	gm

The time to prevent or delay the infirmities of age is before they take over. Abundant good nutrition may be our most effective means of preventing these medical conditions, as well as the wrinkles, loss of vitality and strength, shortness of breath, and disturbed emotional states that all too often—and perhaps unnecessarily —come with the later years of life.

Persons Who Are Ill

Those who are ill (or injured) may have special needs for vitamins. Hopefully, they will be receiving medical or dental care from a practitioner who understands the role of good nutrition in the body's defensive and restorative mechanisms.

Presurgical patients, for example, can derive special benefits from prior nutritional planning, if elective operations are due. If possible, this should be done several months before operation. Several office patients have had special nutritional programs, prescribed vitamin and mineral supplements, and vitamins and calcium administered by injection. One patient who had a pulmonary operation and another who underwent hysterectomy made excellent recoveries and required little time in the recovery room, with shorter and less distressing postoperative treatment. When the patients apprised their surgeons of their rapid recovery from anesthesia and surgery, one received a surgeon's age-old acknowledgment of his own skill: "I must be doing well in my old age," said the surgeon, taking all the credit!

CHAPTER 17:

MINERALS TO MATCH

We know that in addition to vitamins A and C, the other nutrients cited most often as deficient in the American diet are protein and the minerals *calcium* and *iron*. Even when present in the diet, these and many other minerals are often poorly absorbed, especially among the elderly. *Magnesium, iodine, copper*, and *zinc* in particular should also be added, in proper amounts, to complement a vitamin regimen.

The need for these minerals is too often ignored, even by those who customarily take vitamin supplements. But the vitamins often need minerals, either to be absorbed into the body or to be effective after absorption. Among hospitalized patients with known vitamin A deficiencies, for example, high-level therapeutic dosages of the vitamin have been ineffective unless the mineral zinc was also added. Thus a lack of minerals can also prolong a vitamin deficiency.

Further, minerals have themselves often shown surprising medical benefits. *Medical World News* in 1969 described a case, for example, of an elderly surgical recovery patient who developed persistent and severe skin ulcers and sores following her operation. One week of zinc therapy led to healing of most of the sores and an improvement in the healing of the surgical incision as well.

And we have earlier described the value of calcium, magnesium, etc., to general health.

How can one be assured of an adequate mineral intake? Many foods contain a valuable assortment of minerals, of course. In general, these are the foods we know to be nutritious: liver and other meats, poultry, fish (especially shellfish), eggs, fruits, beans, and leafy green vegetables (the outer green leaves of lettuce, for example, not the inner colorless ones). But there is very little calcium in most of these foods. For calcium, one must drink milk, or eat cheese and other dairy products.

But if you want to be on the safe side and keep up the nutritional level of your vitamin regimen, we also recommend a daily *multimineral* supplement, plus additional calcium and magnesium.

For both men and women, the supplemental mineral intake should be as in the list below, with pregnant or nursing women in particular receiving the higher amounts. Older people and large-bodied people should also seek the higher levels, as should those who may be anemic, excitable, "nervous," or depressed.

Calcium	1,000–2,000	mg
Phosphorus	1,000–2,000	mg
Iron	20–60	mg
Magnesium	400–800	mg
Iodine	150–300	mcg
Copper	2–4	mg
Zinc	15–30	mg

The amount of phosphorus should not be more than the amount of calcium. Also, the magnesium content should be a shade less than half of the calcium.

The proposed new FDA regulations are intended to limit the minerals in supplements, as well as the vitamins. Higher levels are permitted only in supplements labeled "for pregnant or lactating women." These are, in fact, roughly the upper levels in the table above, so one way you can get a mineral supplement with these desirable higher levels is to buy such a special-purpose preparation, "for pregnant or lactating women." (Tell the pharmacist it's for your daughter, if you feel embarrassed. It is unfortunate that such subterfuges seem to be necessary.)

Laboratory studies and personal practice show that many minerals are absorbed most readily when they are attached to certain chemicals called chelates, as we have learned from Chicago's Dr. John Miller: Mineral preparations so prepared are called *chelated,* and we especially recommend these, which will combine most readily with proteins for better absorption. So look for the words "chelated minerals" when you buy a mineral supplement.

Many mineral supplements, or minerals combined with vitamins, are on the market, with very little actual mineral content. Be sure to check the quantities. You may readily find supplements in the drugstore or supermarket that are adequate in all respects, except for calcium, phosphorus, and magnesium. If you look at the list above, you can see why. These are the minerals that would be the bulkiest in any pill or tablet. Phosphorus is generally well supplied in ordinary diets—it may often be oversupplied—but calcium and magnesium are often deficient, and these should be in a definite ratio to each other.

Dolomite is the answer. This is a naturally occurring inexpensive substance that contains calcium and magnesium in roughly the best proportion, approximately 2 to 1. Therefore, we also recommend that you add dolomite supplements to your dietary regimen. These can be found in many health shops at very low cost. Enough should be taken for a total of at least 1 or 2 gm (1,000–2,000 mg) of calcium daily. The proper amount of magnesium will then accompany the calcium.

There is no possibility whatever of any danger due to an excess of dolomite. Quite the contrary. While some minerals (iodine, zinc) may cause problems when taken to excess, the calcium-magnesium combination found in dolomite is safe in any conceivable supplement quantity. In fact, this additional supplementation is especially important for the elderly, who may be having bone weaknesses, and also for the many adults whose digestive systems will not accommodate milk and who do not eat much cheese. Calcium is often poorly absorbed, so amounts even up to 4 or 5 gm (4,000 to 5,000 mg) may at times be helpful.

What about the other necessary minerals? Chromium, selenium, molybdenum, and so on? And the salts: sodium, potassium, and chloride? The proposed FDA regulations will permit *only* the minerals listed above to be included in multimineral supplements (after the current stocks of existing, broader-purpose multimineral supplements run out), so unless a court case or a federal law reverses the FDA proposals, it may be difficult to obtain adequate supplementation of these necessary nutrients without a doctor's prescription. This will make adequate dietary practices all the more important.

Many eminent scientists and physicians are preparing to go to court to reverse the FDA's restrictive rulings, as we will describe later. The issue may take years to settle because the Food and Nutrition Board does recognize many additional minerals as "essential in human nutrition." As we will see, the irony of the situation is that the Food and Drug Administration claims to draw its scientific knowledge from the Food and Nutrition Board's findings!

But at present, for an individual seeking better health, let us summarize our mineral recommendations as follows:

● A daily multimineral supplement of *chelated* minerals for both men and women. Except for calcium, phosphorus, and magnesium, the amounts should be as listed above, preferably at the higher ends of the scale, especially for pregnant or lactating women. Other minerals in the supplement will make it all the more desirable. (The larger amounts of calcium, phosphorus, and magnesium needed by the body are often omitted from multipurpose mineral supplements because they would make the tablets too bulky.)

• An additional supplementation of *dolomite* for calcium and magnesium, to bring the total daily calcium supplementation up to at least 1,000–2,000 mg (1 to 2 gm) or more. This will automatically also provide the proper amount of magnesium. (It is almost never necessary to take additional phosphorus because this mineral is generally oversupplied in our regular food. This is the cause, in fact, of many calcium deficiencies—an excess of phosphorus causes the body to lose calcium.)

If you follow these two recommendations you will be insured an adequate supply of the most necessary minerals. Good dietary practices will supply the remainder.

CHAPTER **18**:

An Easy-to-Follow Nutritional Program and Some Advice on Weight Control

Nutritional advice comes to us constantly from all sides—books, magazine articles, newspaper columns, and even television programs. It seems everybody has something to say about food, and we are continually deluged with different opinions and comments in a general turmoil of disagreement and confusion.

Those who give nutritional advice are often unaware that they are attempting to apply to the whole world those special food practices that really suit only their own body chemistries, not those of other people. This is the way food faddism is born. One writer whose body takes kindly to whole grains will extol the virtues of wheat germ for all. Another who likes milk and dairy products will base a universal dietary system on these foods, ignoring the fact that others may not respond well to such a diet. Rare meat, fresh fruit, blackstrap molasses, cider vinegar—each may have its ardent enthusiasts.

Some writers have weak digestive secretions, so they propose foods that are "easily digestible." Others whose systems produce an abundance of digestive enzymes and acids may find such foods causing unease and distress. The fact is that soft-boiled eggs are good for some, but hard-boiled eggs are better for others. Stressing any sort of limited diet or special foods for *all* people is a denial of what we have called the biochemical rights of individuals.

229

Fortunately, however, there are some beneficial food and eating practices that do apply to everybody, even though we are, as individuals, such different and distinctive people. Not only will they improve your health and disposition—you will probably find them pleasant and enjoyable as well. Another bonus: These five easy-to-follow rules are also likely to reduce overweight in a measured and safe way, without stressing any onerous form of dieting.

• First, *include some (complete) protein in every meal or snack.* This should be a "complete" protein, not gelatin (which has very little nutritional value) or another artificial or limited foodstuff. We know that in meals, complete protein can come from fish, poultry, red meat, organ meat, eggs, and dairy products. Combinations of foods from vegetable sources, such as corn or rice (or other grains) with beans, provide complete protein. Nuts and dairy products are a protein-nutritious combination, as are macaroni (high-protein type) and cheese.

What about snacks? Fruit and cheese is a tasty and healthful union, being also the traditional dessert in many parts of Europe. Raw nuts are filling and contain protein—add milk or cheese to complete it. Soybeans are another possibility: Many new types of soybean snacks are now being sold in ready-to-eat form—check the health foods section in your supermarket. Yogurt is another protein-rich snack, which also stimulates the growth of desirable intestinal flora.

If you are a homemaker or cook, valuable guides to boosting your protein intake can be found in several sensible (and even entertaining) nutrition books. We can recommend Linda Clark's witty and lively *Stay Young Longer,* Dr. Carlton Fredericks' informative *For Good Nutrition,* Adelle Davis' classic *Let's Cook It Right,* and Laura Hayden's jazzy *The Hip, High-Prote, Low-Cal, Easy-Does-It Cookbook.* (Miss Hayden is an actress who opened a café called Opera Espresso to test her high-protein vegetarian recipes, and her book is an extraordinary collection of recipes for snacks, relishes, appetizers, sauces, dips, cakes, pies, pancakes, waffles, pastries, and other dishes—all high in protein and low in calories.)

Research has shown that nearly all people maintain the most beneficial blood sugar levels after eating *protein*, not sugar. Protein helps to avoid levels that are too high (diabetic) or too low (hypoglycemic), the latter being especially common after eating highly sugared foods (due to overstimulation of insulin production, called reactive hypoglycemia). Extra energy and cheerfulness, even improved mental performance, results from our first rule, which also aids in delaying those signs of aging—skin wrinkles, loss of elasticity in the tendons and connective tissue, and so on—due to protein lack.

There is one exception to our general rule of protein in every meal or snack. This is the quick snack consisting of a single piece of fresh fruit (but even this would be better—more healthful and filling—with cheese added to it).

• Second, *eat some breakfast every day, plus two other meals, and snacks whenever you are hungry.*

If you are not hungry when you awaken or if you find food hard to take in the morning, try nibbling on a piece of cheese or a meat leftover in the refrigerator. No law says breakfast must be cereal, eggs, pancakes, or toast. Be free to eat what turns you on, especially at breakfast, and what your digestive system likes.

Orange juice, toast, and coffee is a bad breakfast because of the lack of protein and the abundance of carbohydrates. Doughnuts or other pastries are equally poor. This sort of breakfast is likely to lower your blood sugar and leave you tense and irritable throughout much of the day.

Those who are overweight or who ate heavily late the night before are least likely to have an appetite in the morning. If this description fits you, have a small snack for breakfast, but make sure it is mostly protein. Try a slice of cheese or a sausage with that (preferably caffein-free) coffee, and you'll likely feel better all day.

If you are a cereal eater for breakfast, then you should be eating a whole grain cereal, without added preservatives or coloring matter, not the most heavily advertised starchy-sugary junk that rots the teeth, bloats the body, and adds to our national nervousness and ill health. Many new types of nutritious whole grain breakfast cereals are now available, some from Switzerland and others made in America, including some of the tasty granola types.

It's easy to tell which cereals are worthwhile. Lift the box or package. If it feels light and insubstantial, then you are buying mostly air. The nutritious cereals have a weight and heft to them indicating the presence of solid and nourishing ingredients. Also, check the label for the presence of artificial additives and avoid those with added sugar or preservatives (including BHA and BHT) and colorings.

"Vitamin-enriched" cereals are usually no bargain, nor are they notably nutritious. Most are like vitamin-sprayed sugar candy, but at an exorbitant price. One breakfast cereal, for example, called "one of the biggest gyps in the marketplace" by nutrition expert and microbiologist Michael Jacobson, is made from the company's regular line of cornflakes by spraying a twelve-ounce box with a half-cent's worth of vitamins. "At the store you pay about 20c more for that half-cent's worth of vitamins," according to Dr. Jacobson. More important, these vitamins are being added to denuded and devitalized foods, and many important vitamins or minerals are still often lacking after the fortification. The broad range of trace nutrients in the original grain is sadly shrunken in these "enriched" foods. Avoid them if you can.

Breakfast meats with preservatives, especially the cancer-producing sodium nitrite (found in many smoked and cured meats, including bacon, ham, and some types of sausages) should also be avoided. Sausage meat without sodium nitrite is now available from several national manufacturers and should always be your choice.

One of the best foods for breakfast that cannot be well preserved without refrigeration is wheat germ. This is an "additive" that you yourself can sprinkle on other cereals or use with other foods (as a breading for meat, for example) because of its interesting, crunchy, nutlike flavor, as well as its nutritional value. But the most tasty type cannot be found as a packaged food on a shelf, in a jar or box, because it is perishable. It can be found only in the refrigerated section in many health food shops. (Despite its perishability, it will last for weeks in your refrigerator, too.) If you try this once, you will probably find it much to your liking.

After breakfast, what? Almost all people have more pep and better spirits if they eat whenever they are hungry, snacking often with protein-containing foods, rather than eating one or two large meals with nothing in-between. Mother was, in fact, wrong when she forbad us to eat between meals. Our cells need nourishment twenty-four hours a day. Frequent snacking keeps the digestive system operative, maintains a continual supply of fresh nutrients to the body, and helps keep the sugar and fat at optimum levels in the bloodstream. And it also helps in avoiding overeating at infrequent meals, which often accompanies or causes overweight!

• Third, *try to eat at least one piece of fresh fruit daily, preferably more.*

Whole fresh fruit contains natural enzymes, vitamins, minerals, valuable sugars and acids, and roughage.

If you have not been a fruit eater, start slowly with the fruits you like best—bananas and oranges perhaps. The thick-skinned oranges are easily peeled (but leave some white pulp around the sweet and juicy interior) and indeed delicious, not to mention nutritious. *The pulp is also healthful, being a good source of the "bioflavonoids," so-called vitamin P.*

Fruit juices, though often also healthful, are not a substitute for whole fruit. They lack roughage and many other important constituents of whole fruit. Also, juices are more fattening: A glass of orange or apple juice has twice as many calories, or more, as a whole orange or apple.

Some fruit foods seem universally popular, even to those who ordinarily avoid fruit. Luckily some of the most liked are also among the best foods. Melons, in particular, are amazingly nutritious, containing vitamins and minerals in abundance. Watermelons, honeydew, cantaloupe, and the less common kinds are all such valuable foods.

Should there be, however, a particular fruit that "does not agree with you," then *do not eat it,* no matter how much it is recommended for its nutritional value. Many people are "allergic" to particular fruits, and for some individuals, these chemical antagonisms can be severe, causing rashes, gastric upsets, or even serious mental conditions. Trust the biochemical wisdom of your body and avoid those fruits.

But fresh fruit that your system does find agreeable is good in snacks, in salads, with breakfast, and as a dessert. From the great variety now available, find the fruits that are good for you and you will be pleasantly surprised at the toning up of your digestive system they produce. You may also benefit in general vitality and improved muscle tone, skin and hair condition.

• Our fourth easy-to-follow rule is to *eat, whenever possible, natural and unrefined foods, rather than processed and refined or artificial foods.*

It took millions and millions of years for nature to evolve the marvelously complex biochemical system that is man. This evolution took place as a delicate chemical interaction with the external environment. Man was "created," so to speak, to be in harmony with the naturally occurring foods of the earth.

But today, after only a few decades of chemical and nutritional knowledge, many think the natural abundance of nutrients in unrefined and unprocessed foods can be surpassed by our newly found manufacturing methods.

"Technology that tops nature."

"Takes nature further."

"Flavors that nature envies."

"Add more tang, tingle, zip, zap, pep, pop, flavor, savor, gusto, smack, relish, and yum to anything you make to eat."

Above are some of the actual slogans displayed at the thirty-third annual convention of the Institute of Food Technologists in 1973, attended by some 7,000 experts in artificial foods, each seeking bigger and better profits. Newspaper reporter Colman McCarthy commented drolly: "It is as though these companies were announcing themselves as neo-naturalists, that the Second Creation had come and that in the new Garden of Eden stands a tree from which the Almighty Chemists hang the temptation of a fake apple."

Even a former president of the food chemists' organization, George F. Stewart, now with the University of California at Davis, was distressed by the bizarre new artificial foods being exhibited in 1973, stating: "I worry about it. I think it's awful. I don't know where it is taking us. There's a lot of stuff being put on the market that's not food. I worry whether my kids and I will be able to get good food. We may be losing a social and cultural good. But I'm in the minority."

Those who wish to be healthy will have to act in self-defense. We cannot go all the way back to nature and eat raw foods as primitive men and women did (which is one reason why vitamins are necessary), but we can try to avoid the food polluters by selecting natural and wholesome foods in place of the processed and refined ones. By avoiding the artificial snack items—pop tarts, breakfast squares, instant meals, soda pop, sugared and starchy cereals, frozen dinners and the like—we can try to push the big food companies in the direction of distributing foods closer to those of nature, which man was evolved to be nourished by. Some of these companies are already getting the message of this new movement for wholesome food. Have you noticed that some companies are now advertising "No Artificial Preservatives" and "Pure and Wholesome"? The voice of the people *can* be heard.

Remember, eat less of what you know has been mangled, processed, dehydrated, minced, squeezed, fortified, extruded, reconstituted, colored, flavored, waxed, sweetened, emulsified, preserved, acidified, thickened, lightened, or otherwise counterfeited by the food chemists, for the sake of your own body and mind. Avoid those who are fooling around with Mother Nature. Truth to tell, she cannot be fooled. Take her as she is—she's better that way.

• Our last food rule may sound unnecessary, but it is most important: *Try to enjoy your eating.*

In practice, this means you will eat slowly enough to taste and savor your food, that you will avoid eating things that don't agree with your system, and that you will be venturesome in trying new foods.

Many people who think of themselves as gourmets or great eaters are actually cheating themselves out of much of the pleasure of food. Overweight people in particular often bolt their meals—in fact, they often skip breakfast, have tiny lunches, and then sit down to massive dinners, gorging themselves rapidly, but not taking the time to enjoy what they are eating. Rather than eating slowly enough to savor their meals fully, they are filling their stomachs, often rapidly and voraciously, to create an internal sensation of fullness. This compulsion may be overcome by truly attempting to enjoy food —which, of course, means eating often, eating slowly, and *tasting* the good flavors and essences of nutritious foods.

Let us repeat that another way to enjoy eating is to avoid foods that you can *feel* are being rejected by your body. Some react in this way to certain fruits or vegetables, others to milk, others to forms of seafood or meat. Isn't it obvious that no food can be truly good for you or provide any pleasure if your system takes to it unkindly? Gas, abdominal pains, nausea, gastritis, a "butterfly stomach," cramps, constipation, diarrhea, digestive spasms, headaches, and other unpleasantnesses may be indications your body is unhappy with a certain food. No matter what you may be told by any food expert or nutritionist, your own body is generally wisest about your own nutritional needs, as long as it is not seduced by artificial foods. So pay attention to your sensations and trust your internal, inherent biochemical wisdom. Though we all need vitamins, minerals, protein, carbohydrates, and fats in the diet, these can come from many food sources. Choose the foods that suit your own personal chemistry.

The third way to enjoy eating is to be a little venturesome about trying new and unfamiliar foods. There is no reason to be stuck in a rut, eating the same things day after day. In older times, more variety was sometimes forced on people because certain foods were available only at specific seasons of the year. Today, when nearly all foods are available all year long, it is too easy (and too unhealthy) to fall into set and fixed food habits, eating only a limited and repetitious diet. Doing this makes one less likely to be getting a full range of varied nutrients and promotes the possibilities of trace nutrient deficiencies. Switch around. Don't limit yourself. Try new foods, especially natural and wholesome ones. You may find many of them, formerly unfamiliar, to be most enjoyable. And you may also have more vitality and better health.

In summary, then, our five easy-to-follow food rules are:

1. Include some (complete) protein in every meal or snack.

2. Eat some breakfast every day, plus two other meals, and snacks whenever you are hungry.

3. Try to eat at least one piece of fresh fruit daily, preferably more.

4. Eat, whenever possible, natural and unrefined foods, rather than processed and refined or artificial foods.

5. Try to enjoy your eating (by eating slowly, avoiding foods that disagree with you, and trying new, wholesome foods).

Interestingly, many patients who were overweight have slowly and sensibly lowered their weight, just by following these rules and without any other conscious attempt at dieting. Then by continuing them, the excess weight stayed off. Also, they and others have lost persistent heartburn, morning nausea, flatulence (gas), constipation, fatty stools, and other gastric and intestinal distress.

For those who need it, here is one other bit of advice. If you are much troubled by overweight and a complete physical and chemical examination has disclosed no organic cause, there is one further step you can take to lose weight. This requires no "dieting," in the sense that you need not measure calories or otherwise fret about your food. Merely follow the five rules above, with the following significant addition:

Drink no fluids (of any kind) one-half hour before eating, during the meal or snack, to one-half hour after.

By so eliminating fluids with your meals (a practice of most animals by the way), you will automatically lower your solid food intake without ever going hungry. Also, your digestive enzymes will be undiluted and more efficient. Be sure, however, to drink plenty of fluids at other times to avoid dehydration.

CHAPTER 19:

How to Buy and Take the Vitamins
Natural (Extracted) vs. Synthetic (Manufactured)

Vitamins are not found lying around freely in nature like nuggets of gold or clumps of coal. They must either be manufactured, in which case they are popularly called *synthetic,* or they are extracted from plant matter, when they are called *natural* or *organic.* These names are unfortunate and misleading, because a pure vitamin is a specific chemical compound, regardless of which type of chemical process is used.

Synthetic vitamins are actually often made under controlled conditions using "natural" processes—that is, fermentation or cultivation using microorganisms, similar to the way we make yogurt, various cheeses, wine and beer, and other "manufactured" foodstuffs, with the aid of helpful organisms. Thus, so-called synthetic vitamins are not necessarily artificial, any more than yogurt is. A better name for "synthetic" vitamins would thus be *manufactured.*

Many health writers have been misled into thinking that the so-called natural or organic vitamins are superior. Perhaps they are unaware that severe chemical processes may also be needed to extract such vitamins from their plant sources. These chemical processes can be just as "artificial" as those used in manufacturing vitamins. A more meaningful name for natural or organic vitamins would actually be *extracted.*

In many cases a product that a consumer may think is "natural," such as "Rose Hips Vitamin C," actually mostly contains the manufactured vitamin. Rose hips do not have enough vitamin C content to make vitamin pills of sufficient potency, so products with some vitamin C from rose hips must always be standardized or fortified with manufactured pure ascorbic acid, vitamin C, to meet the label claims.

There is no accepted clinical evidence—and we have found none in personal practice—that so-called natural (extracted) vitamins are superior to so-called synthetic (manufactured) ones. In fact, the reverse may be true.

In 1973 the Food and Drug Administration noted in a "Finding of Fact"—with which we agree—that:

> A large number of dietary supplements on our domestic market advertise or otherwise call attention to the claim that their ingredients are "natural" or derived from "natural sources" . . .
>
> More than half of the people in the United States are likely to choose foods for special dietary uses [*e.g.*, vitamin pills] that contain ingredients described as "natural" or derived from "natural sources" in the belief that they are superior . . .
>
> There is no nutritional difference between a vitamin provided by a synthetic source and the same vitamin provided by a natural source, but *the natural source may contain other ingredients which may limit the absorbability of the vitamin provided by the natural source.* [Emphasis added.]

That is, the so-called natural vitamins may actually be less effective than the synthetic ones because they may be less readily absorbed by the body.

Another disadvantage of the extracted natural vitamins is cost. Extraction costs themselves are often higher than manufacturing ones, and in addition, "health food" manufacturers often charge three to one hundred times more for identical vitamins labeled "from all-natural sources" or "ecology" than the price for the corresponding (pure) manufactured vitamin. As Linus Pauling notes, "there is no advantage whatever to buying 'All-natural Vitamin C' . . . or similar preparations. In fact, there is the disadvantage that you would waste your money if you bought them. . . ."

It is, however, possible that there are unrecognized necessary food elements, such as undiscovered or disputed vitamins. If so, they are likely to be found in some food sources—liver, wheat germ, brewer's yeast—that do contain an abundance of other vitamins. Many vitamin manufacturers do include minuscule amounts of desiccated liver, wheat germ powder, and the like, in their preparations. Health food writers have claimed—this time correctly —that the amounts are often too small to provide any meaningful quantity of any of the known nutrients. (How much liver, after all, can one squeeze into a tiny capsule or tablet?) Therefore, these writers have concluded, such elements must just be a sales gimmick to inveigle the unwary into thinking that the product is extra nutritious.

Maybe so. Most concentrated food preparations that are small in size, such as desiccated liver pills, protein wafers and tablets, are indeed nearly worthless nutritionally—and often outrageously expensive as well.

But on the chance that there are unknown and important nutrients that are required over the long term in ultraminuscule amounts, the addition of small quantities of desiccated liver and similar foodstuffs to (already nutritious) vitamin preparations might be useful. The Food and Drug Administration is moving to prohibit them. Until such a prohibition occurs, and *as long as no great additional cost is involved,* one might just as well have the possible benefits of these added ingredients and buy vitamin preparations with them.

But remember that such additional ingredients have nothing to do with the question of "natural" (extracted) or "synthetic" (manufactured) vitamins. Here the decision should always be one of cost, with the weight leaning toward the cheaper, more absorbable, manufactured (synthetic) vitamins.

Fillers and Binders

Vitamins are needed only in small amounts, so vitamin manufacturers, in preparing their pills and tablets, must "fill" these out with other ingredients, then add agents to "bind" these components together in a tablet or add a coating to a capsule.

For example, a tablet containing 100 mg of the B vitamin pantothenic acid or its alternative form, calcium pantothenate, will need about 235 mg of some other material to fill out the tablet. Some common fillers that are used are white sugar (sucrose), dicalcium phosphate, milk sugar (lactose), wheat germ powder, and so on. "Chewable" vitamins often use sweeteners and artificial colors. Coatings, usually a sugar syrup but sometimes made of protein, are often necessary to protect the ingredients against deterioration. Some products are also waxed.

Many people who have a gastric response to vitamin pills or tablets are often responding to these additional ingredients, rather than the vitamins themselves. A large number of adults, for example, are unable to digest milk sugar, which causes them to have stomach upsets.

Should you have an unpleasant stomach reaction to a vitamin product when taken after a meal, pay attention and trust this bodily response. *Change the brand.* Your reaction is almost certainly due to the extraneous ingredients with which the vitamins are packaged, not the vitamins themselves. Another brand with different fillers, binders, and coating may rest more easily in your digestive system. (In particular, we do *not* recommend "time-release" vitamin pills: Weak digestive systems may not handle them well, and they have an excess of unnecessary coatings.)

Buying Vitamins

Vitamins (and minerals) are today available in hundreds of different brands and types from dozens and dozens of companies. The choice is bewildering—individual vitamins themselves, varieties of mixtures of vitamins with and without minerals—and all in varying potencies. Pharmaceutical companies, "health food" companies, and special vitamin manufacturers—all produce vitamin and mineral supplements.

And then these are sold in pharmacies, supermarkets, department stores, health food shops, and also by mail from catalogs.

Sometimes the mixtures and potencies are irrational or misleading. One major respected pharmaceutical house, for example, has a special "B complex" supplement at a special high price, but it contains only 5 of the B vitamins, and some in tiny amounts. Another includes vitamin E, but in such a small quantity as to be meaningless (vitamin E is expensive). In other cases, inexpensive vitamins or minerals are sold in separate tablets, but also in such low potencies that the costs of the fillers, binders, and packaging far exceed that of the vitamins: The tipoff for this is to notice that a 100-mg tablet, for example, costs almost the same as a 150- or 200-mg tablet. Most of the customer's money is going into inessentials.

Mixing and matching these supplements to reach our suggested regimens is not easy. For office patients, an assistant may sit down with lists of vitamin products or get on the telephone to a health food shop or other vitamin retailer, attempting to find as many nonprescription (less expensive) sources for the vitamins as possible. Very often a patient must buy several or many different types of supplements. Having a dozen different bottles of pills and capsules is inconvenient, but turns out to be not expensive on a daily basis, and all things considered, a small price to pay for health and vitality.

As for total cost, a recent study of prices and inflation showed vitamins to be almost the only consumer product that has *not* climbed in price in recent years.

One way to start is by going to a cut-rate drugstore or health food shop (often listed in the Yellow Pages under *Foods—Health,* and there may also be separate listings under *Vitamins*). Most cities and towns now have at least one such shop specializing in vitamin and mineral supplements. When you get there, try to steer clear of the overpriced supplements marked "ecology," "all natural," or "organic." Look around at the various brands and see whether there are also catalogs of vitamin manufacturers available. Many stores will help with personal advice and even direct you to mail-order vitamin suppliers.

Look for the dolomite and general mineral supplements, and also at the multivitamin pills. You often get more for your money with a multivitamin pill, because the cost of preparing the capsule or tablet is spread over all its contents, but you will not get enough vitamins for a complete regimen. You may wish to take one, two, or even three of the multivitamins daily—the limitation will be in not exceeding your desired intakes of vitamins A and D (where an overdose is to be avoided). Another advantage of the multivitamin pills is that they often contain some *folic acid* and *biotin,* two vitamins that may be hard to find separately.

Then, in addition, you can usually find separate supplements of vitamin E, thiamin, riboflavin, niacin, pyridoxine, choline, PABA, pantothenic acid (or calcium pantothenate), inositol, vitamin B_{12}, and vitamin C to fill out your regimens. Shop around to seek the lowest prices. Check the catalogs of mail-order vitamin suppliers and be alert for sales by large drugstore chains. Look especially for reductions in price for vitamin E, which is the most expensive vitamin to buy. The best bargains, in terms of vitamins per dollar, are always in the highest potency supplements. Sometimes these are labeled "geriatric" or "for pregnant

and lactating women." Cut-rate drugstores often run vitamin sales.

One young lady says she goes out to buy *vitamins A, B,
C, D, and E,* so she won't forget any essentials. Of course,
with the many B vitamins, it is also usually necessary to
take along a written shopping list.

We do not wish to minimize the difficulty of buying the
vitamins you need, which is often time-consuming and
frustrating. One reason is that pharmacists, as well as the
medical profession generally, tend to concentrate on
medications for critical care—medicines to help the sick or
injured—rather than healthful items for preventive
medicine, such as vitamins and minerals. Thus the average
drugstore does not promote vitamins as much as it does
cold remedies, analgesics, digestive aids, and so on. Also,
the large pharmaceutical companies prefer to sell such
(often ineffective) medications and remedies because, as
we will later see, these are more profitable and often less
competitive than vitamin and mineral supplements. (Most
of the vitamin and mineral products from the major pharmaceutical houses carry special brand names and are
vastly overpriced.)

It does take shopping and effort to find the vitamins.
Prevention magazine regularly contains many advertisements by mail-order vitamin companies. Write to *Prevention,* Emmaus, Pennsylvania 18049, for this important
health- and vitamin-oriented publication, and to see how
to buy vitamins by mail at low cost, wherever you are.
(Single copies $.70, annual subscription $3.85.) With a little persistence you can usually find most of the elements of
your regimen, and at a cost of pennies a day. At this writing, for example, one nearby neighborhood druggist is advertising (in his window) a sale on vitamin C, with 100
tablets of 500-mg potency for $1.44, less than 1½c per tab-
let. To reach a 1,500-mg daily intake by 3 tablets would
then cost under $.05 daily. Another cut-rate store charges
only $.99 for the same tablets. Such 500-mg tablets are the

highest potency of vitamin C now commonly available (only one vitamin purveyor, a mail-order house, sells 1,000-mg tablets).

An alternative inexpensive way to take vitamin C is to buy the pure *ascorbic acid crystals*, which several mail-order vitamin suppliers and many pharmaceutical suppliers sell, sometimes under the name "soluble Vitamin C powder," at about $7 to $10 for 500 gm. One level teaspoon contains about 3 gm, and this is easily dissolved in a glass of water or juice and stored in the refrigerator. Half can be drunk each day, for a daily cost of under $.03 for a 1,500-mg regimen. The taste is slightly acid, much like orange juice.

Separate vitamins tend to be sold in specific size tablets or capsules, roughly as follows:

Vitamin A—5,000 IU's, 10,000 IU's
Vitamin D—Rarely sold separately. Get from multivitamin capsules.
Vitamin E—100 IU's, 200 IU's, 400 IU's
Vitamin C—50 mg, 100 mg, 250 mg, 500 mg
The B Vitamins:
Vitamin B_1 (Thiamin)—50 mg, 100 mg
Vitamin B_2 (Riboflavin)—10 mg
Vitamin B_3 (Niacin)—50 mg, 100 mg
Vitamin B_6 (Pyridoxine)—10 mg, 20 mg, 50 mg
Vitamin B_{12}—25 mg, 50 mg, 100 mg
Biotin—Rarely available separately. Get from multivitamin capsules.
Choline—250 mg, 500 mg
Folic Acid—0.1 mg (and soon, we hope, 0.4 mg, 0.8 mg)
Inositol—500 mg
PABA—30 mg
Pantothenic Acid (Calcium Pantothenate)—10 mg

Above are the most commonly available potencies. But remember, the specific amounts in our vitamin regimens are only approximations, and slight daily variations are not important. *The main objective is steady, long-term intake of amounts that are close to those recommended, as close as you can get.*

New Vitamin Regulations

Much of the above may change in future years if the new Food and Drug Administration regulations, announced in 1973, are not stopped by court action or legislation and do go into effect in 1975 as scheduled. These new rules are supposedly based on the reports and findings of the Food and Nutrition Board, but, as we will see, they actually distort the judicious and reasoned approach of this scientific Board and establish a framework that could well add to the chances for national malnutrition.

The starting point for the new regulations are the U.S. RDA's listed earlier. The main restriction is that *tablets or capsules containing more than 150 percent of the U.S. RDA's can no longer be sold freely as supplements, but must henceforth be considered "drugs."* What does this mean? Nobody is sure. High-potency vitamin supplements, such as the commonly taken 250- and 500-mg vitamin C tablets or the 200- and 400-mg vitamin E capsules, will become "drugs," to be considered (like aspirin, cough medicines, and the like) by another group, the "Over-the-Counter" Drug panel, which will then have the authority to require that prescriptions must be used to buy them.

The FDA denies that prescriptions will actually be necessary *at present*, except for those vitamins currently restricted, but many are afraid the classification of harmless substances as "drugs" is a step in that direction.

Two vitamins are already restricted to prescription sale in high doses. To buy vitamin A supplements in single pills over 10,000 IU's or vitamin D over 400 IU's a doctor's prescription is now required. (Of course, anybody can take several or many of the lower-potency nonprescription pills, to reach a higher intake.) This does make some sense because these vitamins can be dangerous in large over-doses, but the levels selected by the FDA are far, far below normal therapeutic needs, let alone the danger point. Many have pointed out that the FDA, to be consistent, should also require a doctor's prescription to eat a slice of liver or a sweet potato because these contain two to five times as much vitamin A as the 10,000-IU's FDA maximum!

What about the other, harmless vitamins? Their sale as dietary supplements (no prescription) will be limited by the following table. The middle column in each of the three cases is the U.S. RDA. The rules are complex.

- Any single vitamin or mineral listed in the table can be sold *alone* in a tablet or pill, but only in the amounts within the indicated ranges. These ranges, as the heading indicates, are the only "permissible compositional ranges" for *dietary supplements* of vitamins and minerals."

- Any "multivitamin" supplement must contain *all* the mandatory vitamins listed, in amounts within the permissible ranges. If either biotin or pantothenic acid is included, these being the "optional" vitamins, then the other must also be included. The mineral iron may also be added to such supplements.

- "Multimineral" supplements must similarly contain all of the listed mandatory minerals (within the indicated ranges), and if either copper or zinc is included, then the other must also be in the supplement.

- Combined multivitamin-multimineral supplements must have all the mandatory vitamins and minerals (again in the indicated amounts), and if any one of biotin, pantothenic acid, copper, or zinc is included, then the other three nutrients must be also.

- *No other nutrients can be added to multivitamin supplements, multimineral supplements, or combined vitamin-mineral supplements.*

The first question one might ask is what happened to choline, which is recognized as essential by the Food and Nutrition Board? And what about the recognized trace minerals (chromium, sulfur, manganese, etc.)? And the other *known harmless* vitamins in dispute, such as PABA, inositol, and the vitamin P bioflavonoids? By excluding all of these substances, might not the FDA be gambling too much on the "current state of nutritional knowledge," with our health at stake?

It is true that by requiring multivitamin pills to contain a broad spectrum of vitamins in more than insignificant amounts, the FDA has taken a small step forward. But by forcing the exclusion of beneficial nutrients, it seems to us it has proposed a major step backward.

An even greater backward step is the limitation on the potencies in ordinary vitamin supplements. Linus Pauling, for example, noted that his own vitamin C intake is 3 gm daily, which goes up to 10 gm when he is threatened by a cold. (In a later chapter we will review the vitamin C and common cold controversy.) When he heard that the FDA had proposed limitations on the amount of vitamin C in a single tablet to 100 mg or less, he observed:

> To stop a cold by taking 10 g [grams] per day I would have to swallow 100 tablets per day. I think I would have as much trouble swallowing all of these tablets as I have in swallowing some of the statements made by the FDA in proposing these regulations.
>
> The 100-mg ascorbic acid tablets consist largely of "inert" filler. The large amount of this unwanted substance in 30 or 100 tablets might have some deleterious effect. Also, the 100-mg tablets are expensive—two or three times as expensive (per gram of ascorbic acid) as 500-mg tablets, six or eight times as expensive as ascorbic acid crystals.

In reply, the FDA states it is not removing from the market any high-potency vitamin supplements (except vitamins A and D) or any of the questionable elements (in-

U.S. GOVERNMENT RECOMMENDED DAILY ALLOWANCES (U.S. RDA's) AND PERMISSIBLE COMPOSITIONAL RANGES FOR DIETARY SUPPLEMENTS OF VITAMINS AND MINERALS*

	Unit of Measurement	Children under 4 years of age [1]— U.S. RDA		
		Lower Limit		Upper Limit
Vitamins				
Mandatory				
Vitamin A	International Units	1,250	2,500	2,500
Vitamin D[2]	.......do†	200	400	400
Vitamin E	.........do ....⸳.........	5	10	15
Vitamin C	Milligrams	20	40	60
Folic acid[3]	.........do	0.1	0.2	0.3
Thiamine	..........do	0.35	0.70	1.05
Riboflavin	.........do	0.4	0.8	1.2
Niacin	...........do	4.5	9.0	13.5
Vitamin B6	.........do	0.35	0.70	1.05
Vitamin B12 ...	Micrograms	1.5	3.0	4.5
Optional				
Vitamin D	International Units			
Biotin[4]	.... Milligrams	0.075	0.150	0.225
Pantothenic acid.	.......do	2.5	5.0	7.5
Minerals Mandatory				
Calcium	Grams	0.125	0.800	1.200
Phosphorus[5]	.......do	0.125	0.800	1.200
Iodine	Micrograms	35	70	105
Iron	Milligrams	5	10	15
Magnesium	...do	40	200	300
Optional				
Phosphorus[5] ..	Grams			
Copper	Milligrams	0.5	1.0	1.5
Zinc	do	4.0	8.0	12.0

[1] When labeled for use by infants, a dietary supplement shall contain not less than the lower limit designated for a nutrient in this column nor more than 100% of the infant U.S. RDA for a nutrient ... except that the level of biotin, when used, shall be 0.05 mg per daily recommended quantity.

[2] Optional for adults and children 4 or more years of age.

[3] Optional for liquid products.

[4] Lower limit may be 0.05 milligram until December 31, 1976.

Adults and children 4 or more years of age— U.S. RDA			Pregnant or lactating women—U.S. RDA		
Lower Limit		Upper Limit	Lower Limit		Upper Limit
2,500	5,000	5,000	5,000	8,000	8,000
.....	.....	.....	400	400	400
15	30	45	30	30	60
30	60	90	60	60	120
0.2	0.4	0.4	0.4	0.8	0.8
0.75	1.50	2.25	1.50	1.70	3.00
0.8	1.7	2.6	1.7	2.0	3.4
10.0	20.0	30.0	20.0	20.0	40.0
1.00	2.00	3.00	2.00	2.50	4.00
3.0	6.0	9.0	6.0	8.0	12.0
200	400	400	.....	.....	.....
0.150	0.300	0.450	0.300	0.300	0.600
5.0	10.0	15.0	10.0	10.0	20.0
0.125	1.000	1.500	0.125	1.300	2.000
0.125	1.000	1.500	.....	.....	.....
75	150	225	150	150	300
9	18	27	18	18	60
100	400	600	100	450	800
.....	.....	.....	0.125	1.300	2.000
1.0	2.0	3.0	1.0	2.0	4.0
7.5	15.0	22.5	7.5	15.0	30.0

[5] Optional for pregnant or lactating women. When present, the quantity of phosphorus may be no greater than the quantity of calcium.

* From the FEDERAL REGISTER, VOL. 38, NO. 148—THURSDAY, AUGUST 2, 1973
† Ditto.

ositol, the bioflavonoids, etc.), but merely changing their classification. The high-potency vitamins will be called *drugs,* the other controversial substances are in limbo (perhaps also to be called drugs, or maybe they will be termed "foods"), and then we shall see what further governmental action is to come.

"I've merely locked up your food. I haven't yet thrown away the key," is the FDA's attitude, according to many of its critics. A storm of criticism from every shade of the political spectrum—and from many scientists and physicians—has greeted these proposals. Citizens marching in Washington to protest, bills in the Congress, angry newspaper columns, and nearly a dozen lawsuits are all part of the current conflict. Later we will describe what an ordinary citizen can and should do in this dispute.

In the meantime, remember that vitamins are *foods.* To achieve your own optimal intake, some comparison shopping, trying different brands and types, and daily attention to your vitamin consumption will pay off in better health at lower prices.

When and How to Take the Vitamins

When should you take the vitamins? Generally, vitamins are absorbed best when they are taken with other foods and minerals. The best time is after meals, and as evenly throughout the day as possible. Since the water-soluble vitamins, especially vitamin C, can be excreted in the urine, to maintain a high body level, taking half the amount (or some approximation to it) after breakfast and the remainder after dinner is a suitable arrangement, if it is inconvenient to take supplements with lunch.

If the vitamins must be taken all at one time, then taking them after the largest meal of the day will generally give the best results. Thus after dinner, not breakfast, is preferable.

Since vitamin C often aids in the absorption of iron,

these nutrients should especially be taken together. Similarly, calcium aids the absorption of vitamin D, and zinc that of vitamin A. So try to take the minerals with the vitamins.

The one exception to this general rule concerns vitamin E and iron. These may affect each other adversely in the intestinal tract, so if possible take vitamin E at a time ten or twelve hours before (or after) any mineral supplement containing iron. This way one can get the maximum benefit from both supplements.

But the closest you can come to spacing out your vitamin intake throughout the day, the better. Every requirement of the human body operates on a twenty-four-hour cycle. Your cells do not go to sleep when you do, nor can they survive without continuous oxygen and nutrients. Just as we suggest at least three meals daily, plus frequent snacks, so also your vitamins, certainly vitamin C and the B vitamins, are best taken throughout the day, not all at once.

CHAPTER 20:

A *Special Note for Women*

Probably everybody is aware that the human female seems to be biologically stronger than the male—slightly more male babies are born, for example, but within a short while, owing to natural mortality, female infants outnumber the males, and female life expectancy in our society steadily remains ahead of that of males in every age group. Fewer mortal diseases (including heart attacks up to menopause) come to women—and yet women seem to have an equal or greater number of minor medical complaints as men.

One reason may be the prevalence of anemia due to iron deficiency. That supplemental iron is needed by women in the childbearing ages is one of the few nutritional matters of universal agreement.

In fact, recall that the Food and Nutrition Board notes:

> The borderline state of iron balance is indicated by the greatly reduced or absent iron stores in two thirds of menstruating women, and in the majority of pregnant women. It is impractical to supply these needs with ordinary food, and iron supplementation is required. For these groups, it is desirable to increase the iron content of the diet through fortification.

The Food and Drug Administration says much the same thing in its "Findings of Fact" issued in 1973:

257

Many women of child-bearing age, particularly including those who are pregnant, ingest inadequate amounts of iron in the diets which they consume. . . . The iron intake of many adolescent girls and menstruating women is 10 milligrams or less each day. [The U.S. RDA for iron is 18 mg for adults.] This value [10 mg] is consistent with the 1,500 to 2,000 calorie diet of sedentary women. In addition, the iron requirements of infancy and of the latter half of pregnancy are clearly in excess of what may be obtained from a conventional unfortified diet.

These conclusions have been widely reported, and there is heavy advertising of iron-containing dietary supplements, especially directed to women, on television and in magazines. But the most widely advertised supplements often have insufficient vitamin C to boost the absorption of the iron they include, not to mention their other inadequacies. Nearly half the households in America take one or another of these popular supplements, so it is clear that for optimum health, greater supplementation is needed.

In listing our regimens, we have also mentioned other nutrients (vitamin B12, folic acid, vitamin A, EFA, etc.) of special interest to women.

Women on the "Pill"

Unknown to the public at large, there have been a number of lawsuits in recent years against pharmaceutical companies by women who have had adverse effects from taking birth control pills. Among the problems: blood-clotting diseases, impaired vision, loss of coordination, loss of memory, and severe depression.

From a public health and statistical standpoint, the "pill" has been very beneficial. It has prevented many more unnecessary maternal deaths (due to the normal occurrence of these in unwanted pregnancies) than it has caused damage itself. Also, it has given millions of women peace of mind about their sexual relations. But research continues to find a safer pill.

Birth control pills work their effects by hormonal action. Since many sex hormones are related to vitamins, it is not surprising that the latest discovery in this field, from London's St. Mary's Hospital in 1973, shows that half the women who become depressed while taking the pill are benefited by pyridoxine (vitamin B6) therapy.

Depression due to birth control pills has also been noted to go hand in hand with a loss of sex drive. *Lancet,* a British medical journal, has now recommended supplementary pyridoxine be given to *all* women on the pill. At least half of those formerly affected should lose their depression and regain their interest in sex via this vitamin supplementation. The dosages in our suggested regimens are ample to have this beneficial effect: The other vitamins may also aid in counteracting additional adverse hormonal effects, especially vitamins C and D.

Pregnancy and Lactation

"Eating for two," whether one is pregnant or lactating (nursing), obviously creates greater vitamin needs. Peasant women have known this commonsense fact since time immemorial.

Yet the American medical fad in recent decades has been to stress that pregnant women should not gain much weight during pregnancy. To achieve this, doctors have often put women on a standard pregnancy regimen of diuretic pills (which induce urination and thereby cause water loss, driving salt and fluids from the body), and a low-salt, low-calorie, low-protein diet. In many cases, a reduced—and insufficient—vitamin intake has been a consequence.

Perhaps one result is the great downward slide in our world standing in infant mortality, so that we now rank in this measure of health behind many other less prosperous and less "advanced" nations. Another damaging indication of the fallacies of this medical practice is the rise of low-birth-weight babies—babies born small and puny, more prone to many diseases and congenital defects.

Studies clearly show that a mother who is starved during pregnancy will also be starving her unborn child. Similarly, nursing mothers need extra nutrients if their infants are to be well nourished.

"The trouble is," says Dr. Thomas H. Brewer, an obstetrician and gynecologist at the Richmond (California) Health Center, "there's no money in nutrition. The drug companies want to sell their drugs; it's a million dollar business. And the doctors mostly just want to be able to write the woman a prescription and get the hell out of there and on to their next patient. Nobody bothers to check up on the *results*—the babies produced as the end result of these inadequate starvation diets, combined with the use of diuretics designed to rob the mother of salt, which is an essential nutrient, particularly during pregnancy!

"There isn't a farmer or cattle grower in this country who doesn't understand the need for salt in the diet of a pregnant animal—so much so that they always have blocks of salt available for pregnant cows to lick up. In nature, all mammals do the same thing; they head for the salt lick any time they get the chance. . . ."

A proper intake of vitamins, salts and other minerals, and protein is vital if a fully healthy, vigorous, trouble-free baby is to be produced. Several office patients on the vitamin regimens and dietary practices we are proposing (with no restrictions on fluid or salt intake, and no artificial diuretics since vitamin C is an effective yet gentle "natural" diuretic and pyridoxine relieves edema) have given birth to strong and good-looking babies with *a full head of hair,* a distinctive sign of good nutrition and health.

Our vitamin and mineral proposals (with the minerals at

the upper levels of suggested intake) should be sufficient in normally healthy cases for all the supplementary nutrition needed in pregnancy and lactation, if our recommended nutritional practices are also followed. By contrast, as Irwin Stone points out in *The Healing Factor: Vitamin C Against Disease,* the U.S. RDA's would seem to be far too low.

Notice, he states, that the U.S. RDA for normal adult females is only 60 mg of vitamin C, whether pregnant, lactating, or not. A normal nursing mother will produce 500 to 1,000 milliliters (ml) of breast milk daily (about a pint to a quart), which should contain about 4 mg of vitamin C per 100 ml.

> This adds up to an additional burden on the mother of 20 to 40 milligrams of ascorbic acid a day which is excreted for the nourishment of the baby. If the lactating mother is only getting a total of 60 milligrams of ascorbic acid a day, this extra load leaves her only 20 to 40 milligrams of ascorbic acid daily for her own hard-working physiology . . . [which is far] less than is recommended for a nonlactating female. Draw your own conclusions.

In addition to vitamin C, there is renewed interest in pyridoxine, not only as a counteragent to the common nausea of pregnancy, but also to aid in overcoming the more dangerous toxemia and severely threatening eclampsia (convulsions and coma) that sometimes arise. Dr. Ellis describes many cases of relief of edema, transitory paralysis, the "dropping of objects," numbness and tingling, convulsive seizures, and the like in pregnant women, via pyridoxine (and sometimes magnesium) therapy. And we have earlier remarked about Dr. Luhby's findings of widespread maternal folic acid deficiencies that may be passed on to the unborn child. Pregnant women today definitely need supplemental vitamins.

The crusading Dr. Brewer again:

Then many doctors say that birth defects are a genetic problem. They say that poor people are genetically defective, and therefore are on the bottom of society, producing genetically inferior children. It's basically a racist idea. But we have all this evidence that the most common cause of defective children is malnutrition. It happens that poor people throughout the world are more malnourished.

But not only the poor suffer. Also,

large numbers of middle-class and upper-class women are given the wrong information by their doctors. In their obsession with weight control, doctors often create a state of semi-starvation among their more well-heeled clients. The women obediently starve themselves in the midst of plenty, dose themselves regularly with poisonous drugs which interfere with the normal, precise, delicate, beautiful, physiological mechanisms of pregnancy, and they produce sickly, underweight babies.

For the best possible infant and maternal health, vitamins, minerals, salts, and proteins should all be abundantly present in the diet. These nutrients, not drugs, are the best way to have strong and vigorous mothers and babies.

CHAPTER 21:

The Great Vitamin C and Common Cold Controversy

The public was avid in its interest—and the medical profession a bit nettled—when the distinguished biochemist and Nobel prize-winner Linus Pauling published a brief but compelling book, *Vitamin C and the Common Cold,* in 1970. It soon became a widely discussed best-seller, and millions of Americans began taking vitamin C in such amounts that some drugstores at first reported a run on their stocks.

He and his wife had begun a high-level vitamin C regimen some years before, Professor Pauling related, following the suggestion of Irwin Stone, another biochemist who had long been convinced of its value. "We noticed an increased feeling of well-being, and especially a striking decrease in the number of colds that we caught, and in their severity," Pauling wrote in the very first paragraph of this influential book.

From these personal beneficial effects, he was led to examine the evidence about the value of vitamin C (ascorbic acid). This was more commonly used for sniffles and colds in Europe than in the United States. Many people here, he found, did believe that ascorbic acid did prevent or alleviate colds, but most physicians did not.

Some experiments done in the past seemed to show that this vitamin was in fact helpful to cold sufferers, but none of this evidence was clear-cut—in one case, a large-scale trial, using small vitamin C supplements, had produced statistical evidence for benefit so slight, Pauling felt, that it had been overlooked by the investigators themselves and the medical profession generally. But the evidence was nonetheless there, he claimed, and larger doses would have produced more significant results.

In another experiment, a Swiss doctor, G. Ritzel, had tested 279 ski students. Half got 1,000 mg (1 gm) of vitamin C daily; the other half got a similar-appearing fake pill with no significant contents, which is called a placebo (pronounced plass-EE-bow).

This study was "double-blind," which means that neither the subjects themselves nor the scientific investigators knew who got which pills, the real ones or the fakes, until it was over. (In a double-blind experiment, the pills and subjects are coded, and this code is kept by an outsider until all the data are collected; then the code is released so the results, already fixed, can be tabulated.) This procedure is followed in the best experiments to eliminate the effects of suggestion or wishful thinking by either the subjects or the researchers.

Dr. Ritzel's experiment had showed vitamin C produced a definite reduction in the frequency of colds and an even greater reduction (60 percent) in total days of illness among the skiers. But this study was felt by many to be inconclusive for several reasons. The group tested was small and **not a representative cross section** of the population. Each subject had only been involved **for a short time,** just one week. Also, other studies had not always been able to duplicate such good results.

Pauling also mentioned the work of two practicing physicians in the United States who separately had become convinced of the cold preventive and curative powers of vitamin C in their work with many patients. Dr. E. Régnier of Salem, Massachusetts, had himself suffered extreme discomfort for many years from frequent colds and their secondary infections, until he hit upon vitamin C, which he then found also effective with his patients. And Dr. Fred R. Klenner of North Carolina had for many years used a high-level vitamin C regimen in treating patients with various viral and bacterial infections (and as Dr. Klenner wrote about elsewhere, sprayed on wounds and burns and used intravenously as well, against poisonous insect bites, carbon monoxide and barbiturate poisonings, etc.). Each of these physicians had published his results, but these writings had not been influential.

Also, Pauling noted, others had linked vitamin C beneficially to back trouble (from observations of 500 cases by Dr. James Greenwood, Jr., Professor of Neurosurgery at the Baylor University College of Medicine), infectious hepatitis, prickly heat (for which vitamin C is usually an actual cure), regressions of bladder cancers, general mental alertness and IQ, and so on. No serious side effects had ever been reported, even from large doses of vitamin C. Ascorbic acid is far, far safer than common aspirin —safer, in fact, than ordinary table salt. Although some had claimed vitamin C is linked to uric acid and may stimulate gout, there is not even the remotest chemical link between uric acid (a by-product of protein metabolism) and this vitamin.

Vitamin C and Evolution

Pauling called attention to Irwin Stone's thinking about vitamin C usage in the rat and the gorilla. Under normal conditions, the rat, which manufactures its own vitamin C, produces between 26 and 58 mg per kilogram of body weight per day (and much more under stressful conditions). Projecting this up to man, the equivalent for a normal man would be about 2 to 4 gm daily. The gorilla, which, like man, must ingest vitamin C, lives in nature on a diet made up largely of fruit and fresh vegetation, and consumes on the average more than 4 gm of vitamin C daily.

From such observations, Pauling was led to a bold and

imaginative theory linking vitamins to evolution. Most animals—other than man, his nearby ape and monkey primate neighbors, the guinea pig, and one type of bat —manufacture their own vitamin C and do not need this in their diet.

But this manufacture takes extra bodily work. For the rat, for example, to produce vitamin C within its body, extra labor and energy must be used up. An animal such as man that did not have to manufacture this vitamin would have a slight evolutionary advantage because this energy could be devoted to survival instead.

Primitive man and his ancestors, Pauling theorized, would have had their vitamin C needs met by a diet in which fresh vegetation predominated. This would have produced far greater intakes than modern man receives. And, free of the necessity to consume internal energy to manufacture vitamin C, this would have given our distant ancestors an evolutionary advantage.

Conflict and Controversy

Putting these various sorts of thinking together, Pauling stated:

> The optimum intake of ascorbic acid—that is, the daily amount of this food that leads to the best of health—is not known, and no doubt it varies from person to person. It is my opinion that for most people the optimum daily intake is somewhere between 250 mg and 10 g [grams].

This recommendation was quite at variance with the "official" views. The Food and Drug Administration at the time (1970) used the Minimum Daily Requirements (MDR's), which appeared as the standard on every vitamin product. The highest MDR for vitamin C was only 30 mg daily for adults, so Pauling was calling for an intake from eight to more than three hundred times higher.

The other vitamin quotas, which have now become the single official standard, the U.S. Recommended Daily Allowances (U.S. RDA's), list only 60 milligrams.

Pauling admitted that the evidence for his own recommendation was incomplete. It was based on personal experience and that of his family and friends, on abstract reasoning, and on a careful review of the very few clinical and population experiments that had been conducted up to that time.

A storm of controversy arose. Pauling's high stature as a scientist, the uncommon lucidity of his writing, the boldness and scope of his theories, and the great public interest in colds all combined to bring vitamin C to national attention as never before.

But most medical authorities, including those at the government agencies, scoffed at his views. They were particularly irked by the suggestions that vitamin C was such a cure-all, and they felt that no significant evidence showed it was helpful in particular for the common cold. Arguments flew back and forth over the exact interpretations to be drawn from the scanty research of the past, and the quarrels grew more acrimonious. Pauling had gone over the heads of the medical establishment by writing directly for the public, and this was obviously resented.

Physicians generally have good reasons for wishing unauthenticated medical findings to be kept within the profession and not trumpeted to the public. Quacks and medical charlatans have misled many gullible, misinformed people over the years. Often the real harm is not only in useless and sometimes expensive treatment. People with illnesses that need proper medical care may delay or postpone proper medical aid while they attempt false remedies, often to their later disadvantage. In writing a book for the public—and a wildly popular book at that—Pauling had broken the unwritten rules by which the profession ordinarily attempts to police such abuses.

But Pauling also urged additional experiments and

studies to test these ideas. Other experiments supporting the use of vitamin C against colds began to be reported after 1972—at the Toyei Indian boarding school in Arizona, at Stockton State College in New Jersey, at a boarding school in Ireland, among employees of the National Institutes of Health—but none of these were conclusive. (No toxic side effects were noted in any of the studies.)

The Toronto Experiment

The most extensive and careful recent test of vitamin C was done in Toronto in the winter of 1971–72.

This was a long-term large-scale study headed by three investigators, T. W. Anderson, D. B. W. Reid, and G. H. Beaton, of the departments of Epidemiology and Biometrics, and of Nutrition, of the Toronto Medical School.

Here the investigators, who reported their results in the *Canadian Medical Association Journal* of September, 1972, were refreshingly frank about their initial prejudices and their desire to disprove the vitamin C hypothesis. They wrote:

> *Since most of us involved in the study design were sceptical of Pauling's claims, we aimed to enroll a large number of subjects (1000) in the hope of avoiding an indecisive negative result.*
>
> *Furthermore subjects were instructed to increase their intake to 4,000 mg/day at the onset of a cold, in order that a negative result would not be open to the criticism that we had not followed all of Pauling's recommendations (which include raising the dosage at the first sign of a cold).*

In view of the important and unexpected result of this careful work, let us describe this study in detail.

First, the investigators did achieve 1,000 subjects, as random a group of adults as they could manage, and the trial lasted through 103 days of a cold Canadian winter. Of the beginning 1,000 subjects, 182 dropped out before the study was over, and 28 of these drop-outs are believed due to side effects of the experiment. But these drop-outs were divided about equally between the vitamin group (which had 15 drop-outs) and the placebo subjects (13 drop-outs).

The suspected side effects, by the way, were gastrointestinal symptoms (nausea, cramps, diarrhea), which affected 5 vitamin subjects and 4 placebo ones; skin rashes among 5 in the vitamin group and 4 in the placebo group; and genitourinary complaints, affecting none in the vitamin group and 3 among the placebo subjects.

After the drop-outs were removed from the test results, 818 subjects were left, 407 being the vitamin subjects and 411 the placebo, or control, group. At the end, each of these was asked whether there were any "unusual symptoms" during the time he or she took the tablets—12 percent of the experimental group said Yes, as did 11 percent of the placebo group, so there was no difference here either.

Great care had been taken to formulate a placebo tablet that looked, smelled, and tasted like the vitamin C one. Another trial, when the main study was over, showed that the subjects could not tell one tablet from the other.

Checking against any other possible flaws, the researchers wondered whether many of the subjects could have begun the experiment on a diet that was, by conventional standards, already deficient in vitamin C. Such preexisting vitamin C deficiences could also have confused the results. But this was unlikely, they found, since more than 2 out of 3 of all the subjects regularly took at least 4 ounces of fruit or vegetable juice daily.

The major result of the experiment was not a conclusive negative finding, as the experimenters had wished, but neither was there a significant reduction in the *number* of colds among the vitamin C subjects, as the vitamin proponents had been predicting.

The vitamin-treated group did experience slightly fewer colds and fewer days of symptoms of upper respiratory infection than the placebo group. But these differences were small, under 15 percent, despite the high dosages of the vitamin used at the onset of cold symptoms. This was not felt to be significant.

The surprising finding was a substantial difference in *the number of subjects who remained free of illness or need for medical care* during the period of study. There were 232 subjects (26 percent) in the vitamin group who had no days of confinement to the house for illness, but only 195 such subjects (18 percent) among the placebo group. Also, 40 of the vitamin subjects saw a doctor on a total of 60 occasions, while 56 of the placebo subjects went to a doctor a total of 97 times, so the vitamin subjects needed much less medical care.

Interestingly, the beneficial effect of the vitamin was larger for those who had earlier been more prone to minor illnesses or had more chances of infection during the trial—those who usually had 2 or more colds each winter, were in frequent contact with young children, or who often found themselves in crowds.

But the vitamin apparently produced no greater feeling of "well-being," since about 19 percent of both groups reported an increased sense of well-being and 81 percent did not.

The investigators sought to probe deeper into the meaning of the results. The lesser disability among the vitamin group prompted them to ask: "Did the large intake of ascorbic acid exert a specific anti-viral (or anti-bacterial) effect, or was the mechanism involved a non-specific one responding to any type of acute illness, or indeed to any acute stress?"

Their answer:"Our data cannot provide a clear answer to this question, but the fact that general rather than local symptoms were the most strongly influenced, and that different types of illness appeared to be equally affected, would seem to favor a relatively non-specific mechanism. The high concentration of ascorbic acid (and its depletion at times of stress) may be relevant to this question."

In other words, the greater freedom from illness in the vitamin group may be closer to what we have called "an improvement in health" or a benefit to bodily vitality than to a "cure" or prevention for any specific illness.

This also seems to explain in part the difficulty in interpreting other vitamin C studies related to colds and infections. Often there has been no great reduction in the *number* of colds, but there has been a lessening of their severity or of the disability they and other minor illnesses have caused. We ourselves would rather continue to call this *an improvement in health*.

The Toronto investigators noted: *"Our finding that disability was substantially less in the vitamin group was entirely unexpected, and may have important theoretical and practical consequences."*

Irwin Stone and Vitamin C

In 1972 the man who first brought vitamin C to Linus Pauling's attention, biochemist Irwin Stone, published his own book, *The Healing Factor: "Vitamin C" Against Disease*. In it he expounded on his own theory relating vitamin C to evolution and listed an extraordinary array of medical references, most of which had been generally overlooked, detailing the successful or promising use of this vitamin against many illnesses.

Most mammals are biochemically similar, Stone notes, so it is surprising that so few actually need this substance in their diets for survival. As mentioned above only the primates (apes, monkeys, and man), the guinea pig, and one rare species of bat have this need. Vitamin C has a structure as a chemical molecule very similar to that of the common sugar glucose, and is easily made from glucose in all other mammals and all birds (that is, all other warm-blooded animals).

Stone theorizes that the inability to make vitamin C arose from genetic mutations in the distant evolutionary ancestors of the modern guinea pig, the single species of bat, and the common forerunner of the primate family (which includes man). But, in contrast to Pauling, he sees this mutation as a *disadvantage* today, one that works to create less general health and more disease.

To support this idea—and make a general plea for greater medical use of vitamin C—Stone has compiled an extensive list of medical and scientific references where vitamin C was applied beneficially to many apparently unrelated diseases. These include viral infections (colds, poliomyelitis, hepatitis, herpes, virus pneumonia, measles, mumps, encephalitis, influenza, smallpox, rabies, infectious mononucleosis), bacterial infections (diphtheria, typhoid fever, tuberculosis, pneumonia, pertussis, or whooping cough, leprosy, dysentery), rickettsial diseases (typhus, tick fever, trench fever), cancer, cardiovascular disease, arthritis, rheumatism, allergies, asthma, eye conditions (glaucoma, cataracts, retinal detachment), ulcers, kidney and bladder diseases, diabetes and hypoglycemia, chemical stresses (poisons, toxins), physical stresses (burns, bone fractures, heat, cold, high altitude, wounds, shock, radiation), mental or behavioral diseases, aging, and so on.

The reason for so many possible benefits of vitamin C, he asserts, is that it is not a true vitamin at all. That is, ascorbic acid is a substance that should be in the human body in high concentration, but is lacking only due to an unfavorable mutation of a liver enzyme, an accident of evolution. This is why ascorbic acid can be related to so many and such diverse physical and mental diseases. A high intake (several grams a day) of this life-enhancing substance is the only way for us to overcome this evolutionary error, Stone believes, and generally improve total health.

Recent Findings

The vitamin C and common cold story is not over. In January, 1974, Dr. Brian Sabiston of the Canadian Defense

Research Board reported on a new trial that showed the incidence of colds among Canadian soldiers was cut by more than half when they took high daily doses of vitamin C during maneuvers.

Two groups of 56 soldiers on two-week maneuvers were compared. The first took 1 gram of ascorbic acid daily (500 mg at breakfast, 500 mg at dinner), while the second group took a placebo. Vitamin C cut the incidence of colds to 10 percent, compared to a 24 percent incidence among those on the placebo.

Two additional companies of soldiers on the same maneuvers received no pills (no vitamin, no placebo) and served as additional controls. These soldiers had a 20 percent incidence of colds in one company, and a 28 percent incidence in the other. Thus their average, like the placebo soldiers, was 24 percent, more than twice the number of colds of the vitamin C soldiers.

The vitamin C group and the placebo group were housed together, 5 from each group in 10-man tents. Of a total of 14, 9 tents reported colds. Of these tents, 6 reported colds only among the soldiers given the placebo!

Medical Tribune World Service reported:

> Vitamin C did not reduce the severity or duration of runny noses, sore throats, and chest congestion. However, "constitutional" symptoms—those most likely to keep someone from working—were reduced in severity and duration among the Vitamin C group. *Headache, general fatigue, nausea, and fever lasted less than one day, compared with an average of 2½ days among soldiers on placebo.* (Emphasis added.)

Later in 1974, Dr. B. D. Rawal and his colleagues at the University of Queensland reported on their experiments with cystic fibrosis patients, using vitamin C to boost the power of antibiotics. A marked reduction in hostile bacteria and improved well-being was the result.

The evidence in favor of vitamin C thus continues to mount each year.

CHAPTER 22:

How Vitamins Work

Strike a match and notice the flame. We can recall from high school chemistry that oxygen from the air is combining with carbon in the match, producing the heat and flame. This is a process called oxidation. The waste gas carbon dioxide is produced, and there is left behind the remaining ash.

A similar process, as we all know, takes place within our bodies. Oxygen from inhaled air enters the bloodstream in the lungs, is transported along with "fuels" to the cells where the oxidation occurs, and then the wastes are removed, carbon dioxide being expelled from the lungs and the other waste products being extracted from the blood by the kidneys and excreted in the urine.

But the oxidation that takes place within the cells occurs far more slowly and at lower temperatures than the burning match. And instead of being all-at-once, it proceeds in stages, in several steps.

These steps are made possible by the presence of special important chemicals called *enzymes*. Enzymes not only make oxidation within the cells possible, but are also responsible for most of the biochemical functionings within our bodies—growth, cellular reproduction, movement (as found in the muscle cells), digestion, and so on.

Some enzymes do their work in the digestive tract, to break down the food we eat into simpler forms. Others are found in the fluid serum of the blood and in other body fluids. But most enzymes work inside the cells in the fundamental processes of life.

An enzyme is sort of a chemical matchmaker, a catalyst. It can bring together other materials, see that they combine or react properly, and then go forth more or less unchanged to continue its work with a fresh supply of new raw material. Since it is a catalyst, only minute amounts of enzymes are sometimes necessary.

Each of the many steps of the complex biochemical reactions that make up the overall totality we call life is made possible by enzymes. The body has thousands of different enzymes among its billions and billions of cells.

What has this to do with vitamins?

Enzymes generally contain two parts. One part is a large protein molecule. The other part, which attaches to the protein molecule for the total enzyme to function, is called a coenzyme. Very often the coenzyme is itself a vitamin —or it may contain a vitamin or some chemical cousin of a vitamin, a closely related molecule that the body can readily manufacture from a vitamin.

It is now known that *most vitamins function as parts of coenzymes*. Thus they help make up the whole enzymes that, in turn, are necessary for life processes throughout the body. (Minerals also often function similarly.)

The human body has an enormous number of living cells—from 5 to 10 billion in the brain alone, and each of them requires these enzymes with their coenzyme or vitamin parts.

These cells of course are organized into tissues—muscle tissue, nerve tissue, bone tissue, epithelial tissue (which forms the skin, and the linings of the blood vessels and digestive tract, etc.), connective tissue, and so on. Then these tissues make up the bodily "organs," such as the heart, lungs, kidneys, stomach, and even our external skin, which itself is an organ with many important functions.

But the cell, the smallest independent unit of life, is the

most fundamental part. Understanding the complex chemical processes at the cellular level is the goal of "molecular biology," the newest and most exciting field in science today.

In molecular biology, the structure and interactions of the great protein molecules in living matter are studied. These molecules hold the extraordinarily intricate details of the "genetic code" in the microscopic genes that determine our heredity. They are also responsible for the rich pattern of enzyme and hormone activity and for the slow decline we call aging.

Explanation of the Clinical Signs

The biochemical discovery that vitamins (and minerals) are necessary parts of many enzymes explains many clinical observations about the whole human body and the diet.

First, it explains why vitamins and minerals are necessary foods in the diet, since the body cannot manufacture these vital coenzymes and it must have them to function. A continuing fresh supply is needed, since coenzymes are slowly "used up" as they function.

Second, it explains why vitamins seem to be needed throughout the entire body—and why the lack of any one can often cause so many and so varied a collection of different symptoms. Skin, hair, eye, mouth, digestive, blood, neurological, muscular, behavioral, reproductive, and other troubles can all stem from the lack of any one of several vitamins. This is because each of these vitamins works on the cellular level throughout the whole body.

Most biochemical reactions are several-step processes. Even simple oxidation is done in stages, which result in a slow release of energy as the fuel, usually a simple sugar, is "burned," or oxidized. This means that several enzymes are required, and thus several vitamins. This explains why vitamins and other necessary nutrients work best together. A whole chain of enzymes, and thus several vitamins and minerals, may be necessary for a complete chemical process to occur.

And this also tells us why the initial signs and symptoms of so many different vitamin deficiencies are so strangely similar. These deficiencies often begin with a general vague weakness and depression, which many people may ignore. Then there may be minor skin complaints —eczema, for example, is common in the lack of several different vitamins. Other minor (though often quite distressing) complaints can follow, such as eye, mouth, and mild neurological troubles. Diarrhea and restlessness may also result from a decline in any one of several vitamins. This is because whole enzyme chains are disrupted if one or another of the vitamins is in short supply.

Pronounced and clear-cut distinctive signs make the diagnosis of any health disorder easier, but these do not appear in the first stages of most vitamin deficiencies —another reason why vitamins have so often been slighted by health professionals.

To repeat, many different signs and symptoms may result from the lack of any one vitamin. Also the lack of different vitamins often produces the same (varied) health disorders. This doubly varied symptomatology is due to the disruption, or dysfunctioning, of enzyme chains. It often leads to difficulty in deciding just which vitamins are lacking and by how much.

Aging and Enzymes

Our entire bodies are originally derived from one single cell, the fertilized human ovum. In the molecules of this cell is all the information, stored in biochemical form, that will lead to the development and growth of the fetus in the womb, and then the living child and adult.

This original cell divides and the cells produced divide again, and then again, over and over, for generations of cell reproduction. The *blueprint* for an enzyme is constantly being reproduced. New molecules are "molded" over and over again, in a successive pattern as the cell division continues.

As this goes on and on, it is likely that minor structural defects will begin to appear at the molecular level. The five-hundredth enzyme down the line may not be as structurally perfect as its ancestor, 250 cell divisions back. The large protein molecules can become distorted—just the way a story is distorted when it is passed from one person to another in a long chain of gossip or rumor. Many believe this to be a major cause of aging, which remains one of the great mysteries to biology.

This helps explain why the nutritional needs of older people become slightly different and continue to change with age. With only a minimal supply of vitamins their less perfect enzymes would continue to function, but less efficiently. As time passes and new enzymes are manufactured to replace those used up, the efficiency would continue to decrease. Since the *quantity* of the enzymes in the body would not change, the bare minimal needs to prevent *overt* signs of vitamin deficiency would not increase very much. But the *quality* of the enzymes would decrease, making additional vitamins more beneficial.

Benefits of Cellular Nutrition

A cell which is poorly nourished may actually have many enzymes without the proper (vitamin) coenzyme part. Enough functional enzymes will remain for the cell itself to function, perhaps for a long time. However, the cell will go through its paces more and more slowly until either proper nourishment is received or it dies. This explains why no vitamin lack strikes overnight or in a day or two, in contrast to the quick manner of infectious diseases or foreign poisons. Many weeks, or even many months, are usually required for signs of a vitamin deficiency to appear. The cells continue to function, but at reduced efficiency due to lower enzyme levels. Then as they decline further or die, different tissues and organs will slowly be affected.

Since the external skin is such an organ, signs of such a vitamin deficiency can soon become visible on it in the form of horniness, eczema, or rashes. Similarly, signs can appear early in the mouth or eyes, where the tender tissues may be especially responsive to poor nutrition at the cellular level.

Certain minimal amounts of vitamins can keep most of the cells going. But these cells will be below par—there are just enough vitamins left to keep just enough enzymes operating for the whole system to function—but at a poor level.

However, when a cell becomes bathed in proper nutrition, many of its enzymes can begin to work more briskly. The normal enzymes are now efficient. Others may be misshapen or deformed: Their protein parts can only with difficulty join with a coenzyme for proper functioning. But with a high surrounding concentration of coenzymes (or vitamins), there is now a greater chance of union to form a whole functional enzyme.

This may explain the special virtue of extra vitamins for the elderly, who often report feeling exceptionally benefited by higher vitamin intakes. Older persons are more likely to have more misshapen enzymes than the young because of the longer chain of duplication, stretching back to the first original "stampings" made at the time of conception and when the body was first formed.

Or perhaps a person has been malnourished in the past. This may have been via severe malnourishment for a relatively short time, as experienced by prisoners of war, or it could have been poor nutrition extending over a much longer period. These circumstances may also have distorted the enzyme structure, especially the protein parts of the enzymes, due to inefficiencies in the chemical reactions producing those particular proteins.

Add now a rich concentration of vitamins surrounding or within the cells, and the likelihood for fruitful union between the coenzyme and the protein part of the enzyme will be increased, leading to more vigorous enzymatic activity. Thus we have an explanation of the "acquired vitamin dependency" theory, based on the known properties of enzymes.

More vitamins thus revitalize whole enzyme chains —which is why one vitamin can sometimes seem to substitute for another.

The value of high-level vitamin regimens and their special efficacy—among those who have suffered malnutrition in the past and also among those who have advanced in years—can thus all be linked together via our biochemical knowledge of enzymes and their functioning.

The Theory of Vitamins

We can summarize these discoveries about enzymes and how they explain many clinical observations about vitamins:

- Vitamins often make up the coenzyme parts of enzymes.
- Enzymes work in chains or systems to perform chemical reactions within the cells.
- The major part of an enzyme is a large protein molecule, whose shape is important to its proper functioning. Time or malnutrition can distort the shape of these proteins.
- Coenzymes break off or are used up, so a fresh supply of vitamins is constantly needed.
- Enzymes are needed in cells all throughout the body, so the lack of one vitamin can produce varied effects in different organs and a variety of clinical signs and symptoms.
- The lack of any one of several vitamins can break an

enzymatic chain, so the same signs or symptoms of deficiency are often produced by the lack of different vitamins.

• Deficiency signs may appear slowly, because the body has enzyme reserves in the cells and some vitamin reserves elsewhere.

• Supplemental vitamins work best together, and in combination with minerals and other nutritious foods, because these tend to benefit whole enzyme systems. (Minerals are particularly important, for many work together with particular vitamins: calcium with vitamin D, selenium with vitamin E, magnesium with pyridoxine, and so on. In some cases a slight vitamin lack can often be overcome by increasing another vitamin or a particular mineral in the diet; this stimulates formation of a total functioning enzyme chain.)

• High-level vitamin regimens can produce an "across the board" improvement in health, especially for those who have been malnourished and those who are elderly—by overcoming their lack of sufficient functioning enzymes or weaknesses in enzyme chains.

Minute Vitamin Quantities for Billions of Cells

The theory above seems to tie together many separate observations in accordance with our best current biochemical knowledge. But one major vitamin "fact" remains unexplained. This is how such strong effects can be due to such small concentrations.

Remember, a full *minimal* supply of all the vitamins together only amounts to a daily intake of a few hundredths of an ounce, as measured against the food and water that we consume in pounds. Even the new vitamin regimens only call for fractions of an ounce. How can such small quantities have such widespread effects throughout the entire body, especially since there are billions and billions of cells? Vitamins (and many minerals) are measured in milligrams and micrograms, and these quantities seem too small, to our intuition, to be so powerful.

There are also other cases of powerful effects from tiny chemical quantities. Anesthetics, for example. Also, hallucinatory drugs such as LSD can produce the most extraordinary changes in mental functioning, even in the smallest amounts. The ordinary street dose of LSD is 200–400 micrograms, but physicians and researchers have noted effects after dosages as low as 20 micrograms, and even here, it is believed that only one-hundredth of one percent of this already minuscule dosage actually reaches the brain.

The reason is that, small as the drug and vitamin amounts appear, they still contain unimaginably large numbers of vitamin *molecules*, numbers large enough to bathe all the cells of the body in the needed amounts. Molecules are so much smaller than our ordinary units of weight (even such minuscule units as milligrams and micrograms) that their number is almost inconceivably vast.

An analogy once given by the famous British physicist Sir James Jeans may clarify the point. Imagine, said Jeans, that you were able to take an ordinary glass of water and mark each of the molecules in it in a special way. Take this glass down to the oceanside and empty it into the sea. Imagine all of the waters of the earth—the wide oceans, the many seas, lakes, rivers, and so on—to be thoroughly and evenly mixed, so the marked water is completely dispersed among them.

Then go to any seashore or riverbank anywhere on earth and take out a glass of water. Do you think you might find a trace of your original glassful? Is that conceivable? *There will actually be, on the average, 100 molecules from the original glass.*

This is why micrograms or milligrams of vitamins or minerals, or smaller quantities, can still reach each of the many billions of cells in the body!

CHAPTER 23:

Vitamins and the Brain: Schizophrenia, Suicide, Alcoholism, Depression

The brain is perhaps the most sensitive and responsive of all the bodily organs. In cases of starvation, for example, other organs will waste while the brain will draw nourishment; the body seems to feed it preferentially. It is also the quickest organ to suffer from a lack of oxygen—a few moments of deprivation and it will irreversibly cease some of its functioning. Its extreme chemical sensitivity (anesthetics, hallucinatory drugs, etc.) is now established beyond question.

We noted earlier that "dementia" is one of the signs of pellagra, which is caused by a lack of niacin. Pellagra exists in varying degrees in many places in the world. It is said, for example, that 400,000 Egyptians are so afflicted, not to mention areas of absolute famine elsewhere. Alcoholics tend to develop niacin deficiencies, and pellagra itself was found in 1971 among many poorly fed mental patients in Maryland in a widely reported scandal.

The mental signs of pellagra can be likened to those of schizophrenia and may be linked to criminal behavior. An extensive study of 1,150 persons accused of serious crime in Egypt in the 1940's by Dr. El Kholy found that 18 percent had additional symptoms of pellagra, including more than one-third of those later found guilty of murder.

Vitamins and Mental Disease

"Dementia" is the Latin word for madness, and it means hallucinations, disordered behavior, delirium, delusions, wildly emotional states, and so on. ("Dementia praecox" is an older term for schizophrenia.)

The mental or behaviorial symptoms we have described a number of times, such as depression, irritability, and anxiety—and the more severe signs, such as the hallucinations and disorientation of dementia—are *indications of the functioning of the brain,* just as hypertension or atherosclerosis are signs of the functioning of the circulatory system.

Pellagra and niacin were the opening wedge in realizing the importance of vitamins to mental health. We now know that in many cases, a niacin deficiency has been mistaken for ordinary emotional instability, depression, or neurosis.

For example, Dr. Glen Green has reported on what he calls "subclinical pellagra," very similar to the afflictions of the Hong Kong Veterans, but without prior known malnutrition. In one case, a formerly bright and normal 10-year-old girl complained of various pains and headaches and began to perform poorly at school and to withdraw at home. A physical examination was unrevealing, but there were signs of disorientation and hallucinations. The girl complained of strange sensations, loss of balance, and so on.

Dr. Green began a treatment based on a daily intake of 1 gram (1,000 mg) of niacin. (The U.S. Food and Nutrition Board's recommendation is 15 mg daily at this age.) After two weeks, some improvement was noted. After one month, there was complete relief of all of the symptoms. Hundreds of similar cases are now known.

Please do not leap to conclusions too quickly. This does not mean that all children who are cranky, poor students, or withdrawn at home are niacin-deficient. It does mean that in some such cases, high-level niacin intake has been beneficial.

Nor should this be surprising. We know that many distressing mental signs can be caused by vitamin deficiencies. In other cases, such signs may be responses to deleterious substances taken in the diet or produced within the body itself.

In 1884 J. W. L. Thudichum, the father of brain chemistry, wrote: "Many forms of insanity are unquestionably the external manifestations of the effects on the brain of poisons fermented within the body. These poisons we shall be able to isolate after we know the normal chemistry to its uttermost detail."

And Sigmund Freud, the founder of psychoanalysis and the discoverer of the unconscious mind, once wrote: "The future may teach us to exercise a direct influence, by means of particular chemical substances, upon the amounts of energy and their distribution in the mind."

And in 1927, when vitamins and hormones were just becoming well known, Freud said: "I am firmly convinced that one day all these disturbances we are trying to understand will be treated by means of hormones or similar substances."

At that time, the existence of many vitamins was just becoming established, and their relative presence in various foods was being deduced from animal experiments. But few vitamins had then been isolated chemically, and none had been synthesized.

The breakthrough came in 1952 when Dr. Abram Hoffer and Dr. Humphry Osmond first began treating seriously ill schizophrenia patients with high levels of niacin, to which other vitamins, especially vitamin C, were later added. As many as 75 percent of these patients regained their health. Their 1966 book, *How to Live with Schizophrenia*, describes this extraordinary improvement, possible only after vitamins became available.

Dr. Allan Cott, a psychiatrist in private practice in New York, is another physician applying vitamin regimens to mental disorders. He recently wrote:

> Like most professionals, our training has led us to believe that one's normal everyday diet contains all the vitamins and minerals required and that anyone advocating the ingestion of larger quantities must, therefore, be a food faddist or charlatan . . . [but] A substantial body of scientific evidence has developed in recent years showing that mentally ill adults and children do, in fact, tend to have markedly atypical metabolism with regard to the essential nutrilites (vitamins, essential amino acids, and essential fatty acids). . . . *Mental illness, usually associated with physical disease, has been shown to result from a low concentration in the brain of any one of the following vitamins: Thiamine, Nicotinic Acid or Nicotinamide* [e.g., *Niacin*], *Pyridoxine* [*vitamin B6*], *B12, Biotin, Ascorbic Acid* [*vitamin C*], *and Folic Acid.* [Emphasis added.]

Take thiamin, for example. We know the lack of thiamin produces the severe neurological disturbances of beriberi. An experiment at the Mayo Foundation also showed that a group given a thiamin-deficient but otherwise nutritious diet soon developed aberrant mental traits, such as sluggishness, forgetfulness, and quarrelsome behavior—all of which vanished when thiamin was restored.

Thiamin, along with other B vitamins, is part of the enzyme chain necessary for oxidation, a fundamental part of our metabolic functioning, especially in the brain cells.

Of course, the presence or absence of substances other than vitamins in the brain may also affect mental disturbances, so vitamins are not the whole story. But they are a larger part than anyone had previously suspected.

Dr. Harvey Ross had had orthodox medical and psychiatric training at Emory University Medical School, the Bronx VA Psychiatric Institute, and the New York State Psychiatric Institute, when he learned of Dr. Cott's work. "I was clinical director of a private hospital where Dr. Cott sent his patients, and he asked me to cover for him once when he went on vacation. I had never paid much attention to what he was doing with vitamins until that week, when I began getting phone calls so much alike that they could have come from the same person.

"It was the same story: 'My son/daughter/husband/wife stopped taking vitamins and went off his diet and all the symptoms have returned.' In all my years of general psychiatry I had never heard anything like it."

He then began treating many of his own mentally ill patients with vitamins and nutritional methods, to good result. But he feels that treatment *after* there are signs of behavioral (or physical) disease is not the best approach. The major problem with American medicine, he too feels, "is that it still is not preventive. And I think this is the major contribution that nutrition has to make. Americans shouldn't be having heart attacks at thirty and rheumatism at 20."

Orthomolecular Psychiatry

Twenty years have now passed since the original pioneering work of Dr. Hoffer and Dr. Osmond, both of whom continue their research and treatment of patients, Dr. Osmond most recently with the New Jersey Neuro-Psychiatric Institute. Among their findings was that long time periods were often required with such vitamin therapy, especially for patients whose illness had existed for many years. Also, other vitamins have been beneficially applied in addition to niacin (at about 3 to 18 grams daily), such as vitamin C (3 grams or more), Deaner (a substance related to the B vitamin choline), and other nutrients.

As we noted earlier a removal of artificial colors and dyes from the diet has also been found useful. Also extended testing for "allergies" to common food elements (apples, milk, certain wheat ingredients, etc.) has produced surprising findings. Many "psychotic" or otherwise disturbed patients are indeed not relating to previous unhappy incidents in their lives or to moments of psychic trauma (as "Freudian" theories would suggest), but reacting to biochemical imbalances within their brains due to damaging substances or a lack of vitamins, as Thudicum and Freud himself had predicted long ago. Often such individuals have vitamin needs for normal mental health that are far above the accepted minimal allowances.

Some knowledge of the actual chemical mechanisms is beginning to emerge. A by-product of an adrenal gland hormone may be one of the "poisons fermented within the body" that affects the brain in these cases. Niacin enters into a chemical reaction, preventing this effect of a disturbed metabolism. Also, vitamin C, a known agent against many foreign poisons and toxins, in all likelihood works similarly against internal ones.

A large number of psychiatric researchers have now demonstrated indisputably that many serious mental disorders, especially schizophrenia and childhood autism, and minor mental aberrations as well, can often be benefited or controlled by dietary restrictions and vitamin therapy.

These physicians, psychologists, and biochemists include, in addition to those mentioned above, Doctors Mark D. Altschule, Günter G. Brune, M. J. Callbeck, H. M. Cleckley, Moneim El-Meligi, Masamoto Fujimori, Harold E. Himwich, Robert Meiers, Carl C. Pfeiffer, George Prastka, Bernard Rimland, V. P. Sydenstricker, Jack Ward, and many others.

This work has led Professor Linus Pauling to coin a new word, "orthomolecular." "Ortho" means straight or corrective, and Pauling defines orthomolecular psychiatry as "the treatment of mental disease by the provision of the optimum molecular environment of the mind, especially the optimum concentrations of substances normally found in the human body." That is, the treatment of mental disease not by drugs such as tranquilizers, but by substances normally found in the human body.

Normally found in the human body. This is the touchstone of the difference between vitamins-minerals and most medicinal drugs. The nutrients are needed by and normally found within the body. They are part of life's regular processes. As time progresses and metabolism proceeds, they are consumed—used up in bodily (and mental) functionings.

The newly formed Academy of Orthomolecular Psychiatry, a professional group which held its first national meeting in 1972, is a response to these discoveries. Working with the International Academy of Preventive Medicine, it is providing leadership and information to the medical profession. Organizations including laymen, such as the American Schizophrenia Association, Schizophrenics Anonymous, and the National Society for Autistic Children are also newcomers to the scene, created in the conviction that the members themselves, or their loved ones, are helped by vitamin regimens and related nutritional practices.

And the *orthomolecular* concept—that naturally occurring substances in the body offer unrealized therapeutic potentials—is being applied to other areas of medicine as well.

Suicide

Except for suicide, behavioral disorders do not usually show up in mortality statistics. But the American Medical Association's annual convention in 1972 was told that probably 10,000,000 persons in the nation need treatment for depression. This "depression" is not just feeling sad or blue—it means a state strong enough to affect the careers or personal lives of those afflicted.

All too often, this leads to suicide. Suicide ranks as the eighth leading cause of death in the United States, after (in order) all heart and other circulatory diseases, cancer, accidents, influenza and pneumonia, diabetes, the complex of degenerative respiratory diseases of bronchitis-emphysema-asthma, and cirrhosis of the liver.

Actually the chances are higher that the average individual will be a suicide than that he will be murdered, despite the fact that the murder rate in the United States doubled from 1962 to 1973. Among all young people aged 15 to 19, suicide is the third leading cause of death, and among college students, the second (after accidents). Such a high suicide level is being carefully studied. There is no evidence of any genetic basis for suicide, but it is known that most suicides are in poor health, as can be judged from the fact that 75 percent see a doctor within six months of their death.

Dr. Stanley F. Yolles, former director of the National Institute of Mental Health, believes: "The tendency to suicide is a symptom of a hitherto unnamed psychic disease . . . [which] generally begins in childhood and develops continuously."

How suicide can be prevented is given a high priority in medicine. We know that some mental illnesses caused by organic brain damage (cerebral arteriosclerosis, senile dementia) do carry a high suicide potential. Other suicides are related to schizophrenia. In many cases, both schizophrenics and sufferers from organic brain damage may have their conditions because of nutritional problems. But most suicides, about three-fourths, are either long-term alcoholics or victims of severe psychiatric depression.

Alcoholism

Alcoholism afflicts more than 6,000,000 Americans and is considered by many authorities to be our Number One public health problem. The cause of alcoholism is unknown, but it is believed to be a biochemical derangement resulting from a decade or two of heavy drinking. Confirmed alcoholics do not respond to alcohol as other people do. Once they have a drink, biochemical and neurological reactions are initiated that compel them to drink more and more.

Since alcohol is a pure carbohydrate ("empty" calories in the extreme), vitamin deficiencies of the most serious type can appear among established alcoholics. Cirrhosis of the liver, a major mortal malady in itself, and high blood pressure are also frequent concomitants of alcoholism, which further has been linked to other diseases—stomach ulcer, asthma, diabetes, gout, neuritis, and certain heart and cerebral circulatory afflictions (but not heart attacks, to which alcoholics seem mysteriously immune).

One of the more successful alcoholism clinics is run by the Youngstown Committee on Alcoholism in Ohio. The chairman is practicing physician Dr. Lewis K. Reed, who stated recently that drug treatment was not found to be much help in the work of this clinic. "Only a little bit of medication," he said, was used "to take the rough edge off withdrawal," and tranquilizers were given only very rarely.

"All the commercial houses, all the drug houses claim that their product is the one answer to the problem. They write these fabulous accounts of how their medication will allay the desire and the craving to drink, and I am sorry to say this is hogwash."

Instead, Dr. Reed tells us, *"we take these people who can be treated with a bit of sedative, some vitamin injections, some good food . . ."* and add counseling of the Alcoholics Anonymous type.

He bemoaned the lack of medical education in alcoholism: "The textbooks that I studied pharmacologically spoke of alcoholism in fine print and they would talk about Korsakoff's syndrome and polyneuritis [beriberi] and cirrhosis . . . but actually gave little helpful information." A generation later his son went to medical school, and it was much the same.

Evidence mounts about the importance of nutrition in treating alcoholics. After treatment with specific diets and nutritional supplements many confirmed alcoholics have indeed lost the craving for alcohol and the compulsion to drink. The method is described in Professor Williams' inspiring book, *Alcoholism: The Nutritional Approach*. This is the one disease, he reminds us, in which doctors generally confess inability and turn the treatment of their patients over to a lay group like Alcoholics Anonymous.

One of the two cofounders of Alcoholics Anonymous, Bill Wilson, himself extolled the virtues of niacin, pyridoxine, and vitamin C, together with a protein diet, in the control of alcoholism. He, in effect, attributed this nutritional routine as a major factor in his own control over alcohol. This led him to print a booklet about the advantages of vitamin therapy in the control of alcoholism.

Thus we must conclude vitamin concepts may be most significant in preventing alcoholism and also the suicides that alcoholics are prone to.

Depression

What about the depressions that often lead to suicide? Some of their physical symptoms are described as "headaches, abdominal and back pains, diarrhea, and great fatigue."

Dr. Milton Rosenbaum, head of the Department of Psychiatry at Albert Einstein Medical School, adds:

> Depressions range from the normal changes and grief reactions of everyday life to psychotic states ... The psychological symptoms of [suicidal] depression include feelings of worthlessness, apathy, withdrawal, delusions of sin and guilt, and frequent crying spells. The physiologic signs include constipation, anorexia [loss of appetite], weight loss, dry skin and hair, loss of libido [sex drive], amenorrhea [absence of menstruation], elevation of

blood pressure, and insomnia, particularly early morning wakefulness. One extremely important clinical sign is the morning-to-evening mood variation: deep depression in the morning, lifting during the course of the day.

The similarity between these symptoms and those of vitamin deficiencies and disturbances of carbohydrate metabolism is striking. Recall that reactive hypoglycemia can have a very similar morning-to-evening cycle, and is best treated with a low-carbohydrate no-stimulant protein diet, with many small meals or snacks throughout the day, instead of one or two large meals. This disorder, which involves several endocrine glands (the adrenals, pancreas, pituitary) and the hypothalamus or midbrain, is a glucose disturbance caused by systemic irritability that results in an excess of insulin.

Of course, there are various levels of "glucose intolerance," just as there are various levels of depression and irritability. In some individuals the pancreas will secrete more insulin in response to the same amount of other hormones and dietary carbohydrate than in other individuals. But protein in the diet instead of carbohydrates seems to be beneficial to all, which is why we have so strongly recommended this as part of a general health-building program, with the vitamin intake. Vitamins do not function by themselves but need protein to work with.

The day- and night-time variation in blood glucose has been tested on many office patients in personal practice because these rhythms can have powerful effects on personality and functioning.

Ideally, glucose is highest in the morning and declines after 4 P.M. because of the interaction of several hormones. Persons with low glucose levels in the morning as well as the evening usually are tired housewives or white-collar workers, fearful, withdrawn, and extremely low in energy. Contact with loud and abrupt persons causes inner distress in such persons. They are extremely quiet and, because of their apparent reserve, are liked by all but themselves. They sometimes reach a point where they do not go outside to the store or even to the physician's office unless accompanied by a mate or a close relative or friend.

Persons with low glucose readings in the morning and elevated levels in the afternoon start out tired, pick up speed, and often are better suited to night than day positions. However, their late spurts of energy are short-lived and, in general, pull them down. As a result they are often out of tune with society and their performance is disorganized. They frequently are quick-tempered, suffer from headaches, and are extremely difficult to get along with in the morning.

Finally, persons with high glucose levels both in the morning and in the evening usually are diabetic. Their skin is dry and itchy. Their vitality is low. Their complexion is pasty, their eyes dull, and their ability to function minimal.

All these persons show a disturbance of daily rhythm effects and require changes in diet, exercise, and habits in general in order to establish function in harmony with their overall cellular chemistry rather than in opposition to it.

The powerful effects of nutrition on metabolism thus link together daily personality and many behavioral disorders—alcoholism, schizophrenia, suicide, acute depression, and, as we shall see later, even certain types of organic brain damage due to circulatory diseases. We can then hope that the prevention of such disorders, if not always their total "cure," can be aided by nutritional means.

Organic or Functional Disease?

Where a disease has an identifiable physical or chemical cause, doctors call it "organic." Infections, tumors, anatomical abnormalities, chemical imbalances, degenerations of the blood-cell-producing tissues, and so on are thus termed

organic. Many behavioral (or so-called mental) disturbances can also be traced to physical causes and are also
said to be organic, such as those arising from brain tumors,
cerebral arteriosclerosis, and known dietary deficiences.

"Functional" illnesses, on the other hand, are those for
which we have not as yet discovered a physical cause. Not
only mental ailments, but many forms of illness with physical signs or symptoms are called functional, such as skin
rashes, asthma, and "hysterical" blindness or paralysis.
But usually this term is applied mostly to behavioral disorders. Here the symptoms are more difficult to assess, ranging from minor anxiety and nervousness to depressions
and compulsions, up to hallucinations and dementia.

Around the turn of the century, Sigmund Freud discovered the existence of the unconscious mind. The theory
was advanced that many or most functional illnesses, ranging from the milder disturbances we call neuroses to the
severe and often incapacitating psychoses, were due to
problems with other people, so-called faulty interpersonal
relationships, especially those of early childhood. "Listening and talking" therapies of the psychoanalytic types
began to be used. Gradually, these ideas—at first
ridiculed and reviled, as many new ideas are and have
been—came to dominate medical thinking. Today these
ideas have sunk deeply into our therapeutic practices and
even into our popular culture, and they have become
a new orthodoxy.

The "listening and talking" therapies of psychoanalysis
and related treatments are admitted to be usually ineffective for most serious behavioral disorders, especially those
that frequently require hospitalization, such as schizophrenia, paranoia, manic-depressive psychosis, and so on.
But it is claimed that they are more effective for lesser
complaints: neuroses, mild depressions, compulsions, and
similar disorders.

Many others, however, feel that there has never been
any clear-cut proof of the "functional hypothesis" (that

faulty interpersonal relationships cause mental disorders). There is even no proof, according to the skeptics, that the "listening and talking" therapies provide any benefit at all, even for neurotic conditions. Several studies have indeed shown that merely the passage of time without therapy may be just as curative as the same length of time devoted to extensive psychotherapy.

One new treatment of the past decades for mental disease has been by chemical methods, using various drugs such as tranquilizers and antidepressants for their disturbing symptoms and signs. Such drugs have been used—and often misused—effectively in many cases, but mostly only in a palliative or symptom-reducing manner. Though they do not get at the root cause of any mental disorder, these drug methods have spurred a new interest in chemistry as related to mental functionings and psychological effects.

The newest breakthrough from the methods now called orthomolecular psychiatry means the entire concept of "functional" disorder has to be carefully rescrutinized. It may have been a false direction for medical theory, as more and more doctors now believe. The neurosurgeon Thomas H. Ballentine, Jr., of Massachusetts General Hospital and Harvard Medical School, for example, now states clearly: "What has been shown beyond any reasonable doubts is that psychiatric illnesses are organically caused and can be organically treated."

This is all the more important because an attitude of contempt has frequently surrounded such complaints, especially when they have been vague. Where there were no physical symptoms to be treated or incapacity sufficiently severe to require hospitalization, both physicians and laymen alike have often tended to "blame" the patient. Indeed, often the patient blamed himself. He—or she—was "weak" or "neurotic."

For a parallel, let us go back momentarily into the history of medicine and disease. At one time—and it was not so long ago—diseases were considered manifestations of divine displeasure. Behind the illness of an individual or a plague engulfing a society was the idea of supernatural punishment for sinful acts. Wounds in battle, other physical injuries, and the events of old age may have been considered honorable afflictions, but little else. People blamed themselves, and were blamed by others, for disease. Lepers, for example, were once widely considered morally unclean.

Then, as medicine advanced and it was discovered that filth and unsanitary conditions bred many diseases, and later that bacteria and other microbes proliferating in such uncleanliness were often the direct cause of disease, attitudes began to change. Persons with such maladies were no longer looked down upon as somehow unworthy—they had merely contracted infections. Lepers then became, in the eyes of enlightened society, simply unfortunate victims of a bacterial infection.

Serious mental disorders still often carry the stigma of a moral weakness. But when it is discovered that the afflicted person has been niacin deficient or has a sugar metabolism problem, then he or she becomes a "patient" to the lay world and receives sympathy rather than contempt.

We have not yet reached the stage where medical science can readily treat most complaints of most patients. Muscle and back pains, rheumatism, arthritis, and in addition the so-called neurotic complaints (among them heart palpitations, depression, anxiety, and so on) are among those ills that cannot be "cured" readily by known methods.

Yet there is new hope from many of the recent nutritional discoveries we have described. Special vitamin regimens and related dietary practices are now being applied beneficially to rheumatism, arthritis, and related chronic afflictions, as well as with "neurotics" and "hypochondriacs." Many personal office patients with various ailments have been strikingly benefited.

As such results become better known among physicians and researchers, greater improvements can be expected. Better methods of treatment will be discovered. Physicians will deal more with the "whole" person. Patients with vague or minor mental problems will be treated more compassionately—and be helped rather than scorned. They will also cease to blame themselves, or be blamed by their families and loved ones, for their ailments.

Doctors have often admitted ruefully that more than half of their patients have psychogenically induced or psychologically based conditions at the root of most of their troubles. These could not be treated effectively. But the new orthomolecular concepts, so simple and often effective, may offer the newest promise for both physician and patient.

CHAPTER 24:

Heart and Circulatory Diseases, and the Perils of Homogenized Milk

One of the most vigorous controversies in medicine today is over the causes of heart and other vascular diseases. The human circulatory system is made up of a double muscular pump—the heart—and miles and miles of flexible tubing—the arteries, veins, capillaries, and smaller blood vessels. Diseases and malfunctions of the system can occur in many ways, with heart attacks (technically called *myocardial infarctions* today) leading all lists as our major cause of death.

Atherosclerosis, you will recall, is a condition of degeneration of the blood vessels, often beginning with internal lesions, followed by fatty (cholesterol) plaque deposits which thicken the internal walls. This is believed to reduce circulation and thereby also vitality and strength. A blood clot or floating plaque itself may block a thickened vessel leading to a heart attack or stroke. Or the vessel walls may in time become impregnated with minerals, "hardening" the artery—when this occurs in the brain, it is called cerebral arteriosclerosis, and leads to senile dementia.

Recall also that the lack of a number of vitamins and minerals have been shown in animal experiments to induce one or another of these undesirable states. A lack of either pyridoxine or magnesium, for example, brought about such lesions and calcification of the arteries in test animals. Such findings have only intensified the controversy and mystery of the causes of human atherosclerosis, which now appears in larger and larger parts of our population, and at younger and younger ages.

Animal Fats, Cholesterol, and Heart Disease

On one side of the current controversy are those who primarily blame animal fats and other saturated fats, which they believe should be removed from or minimized in the diet. They point to animal experiments in which high saturated-fat diets, including high levels of cholesterol, have induced lesions in the arteries, atherosclerosis, and heart attacks. They also cite the results of wartime conditions, such as those found in Denmark and Austria during World War II. Circumstances then forced a radical change in the diet. Dairy products and meats disappeared for the civilian populations. Without these rich animal-fat foods, heart disease and related afflictions fell dramatically.

Impressed by this reasoning, the American Heart Association and many physicians have been stressing the need to replace the saturated animal fats in our diet with "polyunsaturated" ones. These are believed to help "flush" the arteries of fat deposits and so aid in preventing circulatory disease. Many consumer products, such as margarines and cooking oils, now incessantly advertise their content of polyunsaturated oils on television and in the mass magazines, and their consumption has risen greatly.

But there is another view, holding that other dietary factors or changes in habits may have been more responsible for the wartime decreases in the number of heart attacks. Less efficient wheat-milling procedures increased the B vitamin content of the grains that were eaten, for example, and also their vitamin E and mineral content. Occupied or war-disrupted nations in the twentieth century also often had a decline in the number of hospitalizable mental patients. Perhaps the additional vitamins and minerals in the daily food helped lower both the circulatory and mental disease rates.

This thinking gains support from experiments in which very high animal-fat cholesterol diets were fed to test animals, some of which also received supplementary vitamins and minerals in abundance. The animals without the supplements did develop a fatty degeneration of the arteries and related circulatory diseases. But the animals who got supplements in their diet did not. They became obese, but their arteries were not damaged, nor was there much cardiovascular disease. The additional nutrients apparently protected the animals against heart disease and atherosclerosis.

Further evidence against the animal-fat theory comes from examining some unusual human communities. Among the Masai in Africa, for example, the diet is mostly cow's blood and milk, which is very high in animal fats, yet there are few signs of ciculatory disease.

Also, the Abkhazian people in the Soviet Union have been studied, because they have exceptional longevity, great physical stamina, and little circulatory disease. (In fact, a seven-year study of 123 Abkhazians over one hundred years of age also disclosed no cases of mental illness or cancer.) These people eat meat, cheese, fruit, vegetables, and they also smoke and drink.

"My confidence in the importance to health and longevity of a low-animal fat, low-cholesterol, low-caloric diet was somewhat shaken by eating habits in the Caucasus," wrote Dr. Alexander Leaf, a gerontologist, or longevity specialist, who has studied the region.

Exercise, Air Pollution, Stress

But the Abkhazians do engage in continuous lifelong *physical labor*, as do most other long-lived groups that are being studied—the Vilcabambans in Equador, the Hunzas in Pakistan, and others. Thus it may well be that a high level of physical exertion plays a major role in preventing fat deposits in the arteries and the circulatory diseases these induce.

But exercise is not the whole story: Another study matched 28 railway men from North India who ate much animal fat against 28 Southern India railway men whose diet had only one-tenth the amount of fat. Presumably both groups had about the same amount of physical exertion or exercise required by their occupation. There were also no significant differences in their blood fat levels, and yet the heart disease rate was said to be much higher among the Southern railway men.

Further, the world's highest known heart attack death rate is held by the lumber-producing inhabitants of East Finland, who engage in great amounts of physical exertion.

Other parts of this confusing picture, and additional arguments against the animal fat and cholesterol theory, come from Roseta, Pennsylvania, where an Italian immigrant group had a much higher-than-average saturated animal-fat diet, but less than half the average American incidence of heart disease. Also, a study of 27,000 East Indians in Kenya showed the same percentage of heart disease among different groups, one of which had a high animal-fat diet, and another made up of vegetarians whose diet was high in polyunsaturated oils.

And there are always the primitive Eskimos, who had the highest animal-fat diet of any group, with their blubber diet. Several studies in the past showed no signs of circulatory or kidney diseases, even among older Eskimos between forty and sixty, ages at which these complaints are common in modern America.

Is *air pollution* a major factor? We noted earlier that those in rural areas have a notably lower heart attack rate than those in metropolitan areas, with the disparity increasing with age. The longer a person is in a city environment, the more likely a heart attack, as compared to his counterpart of the same age on the farm. Since farmers and city folk generally eat the same food nowadays, this potential cause of heart attacks is gaining increasing support among professional investigators.

Or is *personal stress* a major component? This idea is scoffed at by the vitamin E proponent Dr. Wilfred E. Shute, who with his brother Dr. Evan Shute has treated or supervised the treatment of 30,000 cardiac patients. He writes:

> . . . the stress and strain of travelling 60 miles is infinitely less in driving a car than it was in travelling the same distance in a jolting stage coach threatened by robbers and hostile Indians . . . If our ancestors could live on isolated farms threatened by Indian raids and not get coronaries, stress can hardly be bad for the heart.
>
> Overexertion, like shoveling snow after a blizzard, would be a joke to our forebears . . . True, men do have heart attacks while shoveling snow, but for the causation, except for the immediate provocation, we must look elsewhere. . . .

And as Dr. Shute and others have pointed out, animal fats in the American diet have gone down greatly during the past two decades, without a corresponding drop in heart attacks. Vegetable oils, especially polyunsaturated oils, have risen to match, but such oils do increase the body's needs for vitamin E. Most of these oils have been heat treated, and a number of experiments with animals show such refined oils actually promote atherosclerosis.

"The indiscriminant eating of polyunsaturated vegetable oils . . . must be strongly condemned," asserts Professor Roger J. Williams, because "they are another source of danger to the cardiovascular system . . . most commercial 'polyunsaturated' vegetable oils are possibly productive of atherosclerosis and should be avoided by the consumer."

By contrast, unheated and unbleached oils, especially those labeled "unrefined, cold-pressed" in reputable health food shops, produced lower blood fat levels and less severe signs of atherosclerosis among test animals. These oils still contain more of their original nutrients.

Vitamins and Circulatory Disease

Dr. Evan Shute and Dr. Wilfred E. Shute believe that a long-term, unrecognized, and widespread vitamin E deficiency in the United States and Canada is responsible for many heart attacks due to blood clots. Vitamin E therapy is the major part of their treatment of cardiac patients. How vitamin E is related to blood clotting and fat metabolism is still being investigated, but it is clear that pure fat calories, without the fat-soluble vitamins, are just as "empty" as those of refined sugar.

Dr. John M. Ellis in *Vitamin B6: The Doctor's Report* notes that many of his own patients

> had been eating diets containing more than 50 percent fats. When a person eats the fat from a steak, he gets no minerals, no vitamins, no enzymes, no nutrients—just calories . . . A diet composed of 50 percent fat means that half of the diet provides no proper nutrition. The vitamins, minerals, and other nutrients have to come from the other half of the diet. The fat-eater is as bad off in most ways as the man who expects to get his calories from alcohol alone. When alcohol displaces food, the person develops vitamin deficiencies. The same severe deficiencies may come from burning calories from fat—or sugar—alone.

Without the proper nutrients to metabolize them properly, fats in the diet, just like sugars, are then a strain on bodily systems. Thus our circulatory diseases may be more affected by what is left out of our diets than by what is included.

A very large number of vitamins and minerals are now

known to be related to heart attacks, arteriosclerosis, strokes, and related conditions. Included are vitamin A, thiamin, riboflavin, niacin, biotin, choline, inositol, pyridoxine, folic acid, vitamin C, vitamin E, iron, magnesium, potassium, and other minerals. Some of these have been shown to lower blood cholesterol or prevent high levels of cholesterol from arising in the first place (biotin, choline, niacin, inositol, vitamin C, pyridoxine). Others demonstrably improve circulation (folic acid, vitamin E). Still others have counteracted actual heart conditions (thiamin, magnesium) in hospital treatment. Regions of the United States with "hard" water have lower heart attack rates, presumably due to nutrient minerals in the drinking water.

This is why we have laid such stress on vitamin regimens accompanied by proper mineral intake as a preventive practice for good health, rather than merely stressing a lowering of the fat intake. Together with exercise, such a nutritional enrichment of the diet may be the most important preventive step one can take.

After reviewing all the research, Professor Williams concludes that to prevent heart and related diseases, "I think that the evidence points strongly toward the conclusion that the nutritional environment of the body cells —involving minerals, amino acids, and vitamins—is crucial, and that the amount of fat or cholesterol consumed is relatively inconsequential."

Some results in hospitals and clinics with actual patients tend to confirm the laboratory or statistical findings. For example, in California Dr. Lester M. Morrison and Dr. W. F. Gonzalez studied 600 patients at the Los Angeles County Hospital, all of whom had survived heart attacks. Some were given a special diet with large amounts of choline, plus other vitamins and especially nutritious food. This diet was heavy in the often-avoided cholesterol-containing foods—eggs, butter, meat, liver, and so on. Other heart attack survivors did not receive the vitamin supplements and had an ordinary "heart disease" diet (low in fats and salt, low in calories). During one year's observation, there were no fatalities in those on the vitamin regimen and (high cholesterol) nutritious diet, while death came to 25 percent in the group receiving ordinary care.

The Question of Cholesterol

But the questions remain. Is cholesterol in the bloodstream necessarily harmful? And if the cholesterol level is high, is this due to cholesterol in the diet?

The late Dr. Paul Dudley White, one of America's leading heart specialists and a special proponent of exercise, was skeptical of the latter, stating: "The amount of cholesterol in the blood—we call it serum cholesterol—is not necessarily related to cholesterol found in food."

And Dr. Michael De Bakey, a heart surgeon who has studied this problem for decades, wrote in the *Journal of the American Medical Association:*

> An analysis of cholesterol values by usual hospital laboratory methods in 1,700 patients with atherosclerotic disease revealed no definite correlation between serum cholesterol levels and the nature and extent of atherosclerotic disease. Eight out of ten patients had cholesterol values below 300 mg/100 ml, the upper limits of normal for the procedure employed. Associated diseases such as diabetes mellitus and arteriosclerotic heart disease, age, and anatomical location and extent of atherosclerotic disease did not significantly alter the distribution of cholesterol values.

Thus, for example, those who are avoiding eggs, cream, and rich meats are likely to be doing so unnecessarily.

In my own (Dr. Rosenberg's) practice, office patients are regularly tested for blood fat levels. The test results are related to diet, supplementary nutrients, and levels of exercise. High cholesterol and triglyceride serum levels (which are still not convicted as the *cause* of atherosclerosis) seem to arise as often from high *carbohydrate* intakes, coupled with the absence of vitamins and minerals and the avoidance of exercise, as from eating fats.

Cause is one thing—amelioration or cure is another. Here the results of all known medical treatment have been scanty, but there are new, promising avenues. As mentioned above, the Drs. Shute describe many cases of cardiac recovery following high-level vitamin E regimens. This vitamin is known to improve circulation as well as act against blood clots.

Also, *folic acid* was administered to a group of elderly patients who were believed to be well nourished, but who had vision problems. The result was a betterment of vision, ascribed to a greater capillary circulation due to a diminished atherosclerosis in the blood vessels of the eye.

Whether such results can translate into the *prevention* of circulatory diseases remains to be seen, but, as we will describe below, folic acid has been the therapeutic agent in very recent and quite remarkable findings reported by a Connecticut cardiologist and pharmacologist, Dr. Kurt A. Oster. This is another example of the beneficial effects that may ensue from high-level vitamin regimens, which as we already know may also lower blood cholesterol, reduce potentially damaging blood clotting, improve circulation, and thereby possibly reduce the chances of heart attacks, strokes, arteriosclerosis, and so on.

Folic Acid and the Perils of Homogenized Milk

"Is an Enzyme in Homogenized Milk the Culprit in Dietary-Induced Atherosclerosis?" is the provocative title of Dr. Oster's paper, appearing in the November, 1973, issue of *Medical Counterpoint*. Dr. Oster, himself a survivor of two heart attacks and currently Chief of Cardiology at Bridgeport's Park City Hospital, brings impressive credentials to his unorthodox theory and treatment. A Fellow of the American College of Physicians, of the American College of Cardiology, and of the American College of Pharmacology, Dr. Oster has long been unconvinced by the current dogma that animal-fat, cholesterol-containing foods may induce or worsen atherosclerosis.

The basic damaging agent, he believes, is an enzyme called xanthine oxidase. This is normally found in the human body, but only in certain locations such as the liver. It is not normally present at the walls of arteries or at the site of the heart muscle. Xanthine oxidase is present in cow's milk but not in human milk. According to Dr. Oster's view, the xanthine oxidase enzyme can attack the arterial wall or the heart muscle directly, if it reaches these sites. If it is at the artery that the assault takes place, the body lays down the fatty streaks and cholesterol deposits we call atherosclerosis *to protect itself,* just as the exterior of the hand or foot develops a callus (or a corn or bunion) *as a protective measure.*

How does the xanthine oxidase get to the artery or heart muscle? It can come from within the body or externally through the diet. From within the body it would probably come from the liver. This *might* explain one medical puzzle related to heart attacks: Alcoholics are known to have a far *below normal* heart attack rate. Why should alcoholics have special protection against heart attacks, especially when they are extra prone to so many other diseases? Perhaps this is because many alcoholics have extensive liver damage (and hence, possibly, less xanthine oxidase is produced in the liver).

The dietary route (xanthine oxidase in food going into the bloodstream) would seem impossible because large protein molecules such as enzymes ordinarily are not absorbed without first being digested (that is, broken up into smaller and different chemical compounds—into amino acids, in fact). Dr. Oster's startling thesis, which follows some thirty years of pharmacological study (and fifteen years of teaching pharmacology), is that effective xanthine oxidase cannot enter the body from cow's milk via the digestive tract when milk is curdled or preboiled (which "kills" the enzyme), or from ordinary whole milk (the enzyme is in particles too big to be absorbed from the digestive tract). But when the milk is *homogenized*, the smaller particle size permits the damaging xanthine oxidase to pass through the intestinal lining to enter the bloodstream, and then to attack the arterial walls and heart muscle.

As the following table shows, there is indeed a surprising correlation between heart disease deaths and national intakes of homogenized milk. This begins in childhood, he believes, especially in America, due to our high milk consumption.

ATHEROSCLEROSIS DEATH RATE AND FLUID MILK CONSUMPTION

Country	Death rate per 100,000 (1967)	Milk intake (pounds per person)	Homogenized	Preboiled
Finland	244.7	593	About 33%	No
United States	211.8	273	Almost all	No
Australia*	204.6	304	15%	No
Canada	187.4	288	Partly	No
United Kingdom	140.9	350	About 7½%	No
The Netherlands	106.9	337	Infrequently	—
West Germany	102.3	213	Partly	—
Austria	88.6	327	Occasionally	—
Italy	78.9	137	12.5%	Yes
Switzerland	75.9	370	Small quantity	Yes
Sweden	74.7	374	—	Yes
France	41.7	230	Negligible	Yes
Japan	39.1	48	Occasionally	—

* In New South Wales, *all* milk served at school lunches is homogenized.

Note that the French, who are Olympian cheese, butter, and egg eaters, and thus have a high cholesterol diet, still rank close to the bottom of the heart disease death scale.

The xanthine oxidase in their milk cannot be absorbed into the bloodstream because their milk is not homogenized and mostly preboiled. The East Finns have a very high heart disease death rate despite their agrarian life-style requiring heavy physical exertion. The Japanese, at the very bottom of the chart, live in a society noted for personal emotional stress (and much high blood pressure) but their death rate due to heart attacks is surprisingly low. There is an approximately sixfold difference in heart attack death rates between the Japanese and the Finns—an exceptionally wide disparity. According to Dr. Oster, the "biologically available" xanthine oxidase from homogenized fluid cow's milk is the key factor in this great variation. Homogenization of milk became widespread in the United States shortly before the heart attack death rate began to skyrocket, another link between this theory and the known statistics.

To test his theory on individual patients, Dr. Oster first sought an antagonist or "inhibitor" for xanthine oxidase. He began with the drug allopurinol and patients afflicted with angina pectoris. Angina is another puzzling malady: Its sufferers experience excruciating chest pains, especially after exertion, emotional stress, or overeating. The pains are believed due to inadequacies in the circulation of the arteries that supply the heart muscle, the coronary arteries. The usual treatment is via nitroglycerin tablets, which, when placed under the tongue, provide relief in a manner no one understands fully.

Angina patients given the allopurinol to counteract xanthine oxidase soon reported a significant decrease in the amount of nitroglycerin tablets they required to alleviate their pain. This was a tiny step toward verification of his theory. But allopurinol, a synthetic drug, produced harmful side effects. "Because of its potential toxicity in prolonged use, it was not recommendable," Dr. Oster, himself a sufferer from angina, writes.

Instead, he turned to folic acid, which also has the chemical structure needed to counteract the enzyme and is harmless to human beings in any known dosages. For his patients he selected those with high blood levels of uric acid ("hyperuricemia" cases, a condition related to gout and gouty arthritis) and also elderly diabetics. Such diabetics often develop atherosclerotic lesions that are *visible* in the extremities, such as in their toes, and ulcers or sores often accompany these peripheral atherosclerotic lesions.

Certain experiments established that the dosage level needed by a person of average weight should be about 80 mg daily of folic acid (remember the U.S. RDA for folic acid is only 0.4 mg, and the FDA limits this vitamin, even by prescription, to 1 mg per capsule or less).

Dr. Oster writes: "All sixteen cases of hyperuricemia responded well. High uric acid levels were lowered to normal ranges with folic acid therapy, a level maintainable for twelve months. Cessation of treatment resulted in hyperuricemia." In other words, when the high level folic acid dosages were discontinued, the blood levels of uric acid rose again.

The results were even more striking with the elderly diabetic patients who had visible atherosclerotic lesions. "Patients with ulceration and . . . discoloration of the toes were given 80 mg folic acid daily in divided doses. *After three weeks of therapy, lesions which had been resistant to treatment with every known modality improved noticeably.*" (Emphasis added.)

One patient, in fact, as Dr. Oster has told us privately, was in such an advanced stage of pain that he was nearly suicidal. He had been treated at the Cleveland Clinic and at Yale, to no avail. Amputation was being discussed. He could not walk unaided from the airplane to the terminal in March, when folic acid therapy was begun. But by the end of June the patient had recovered sufficiently to be out on the links playing golf!

"These amazing therapeutic responses of hyperuricemia and peripheral atherosclerotic lesions are encouraging," writes Dr. Oster in *Medical Counterpoint* in 1973. "Hopefully, other investigators will try this newly devised therapy with similar results."

It is too early to tell whether this treatment will have the wide applicability it seems to promise, and whether folic acid will also be found effective as a preventive procedure, to inhibit the onset of atherosclerosis, heart diseases, strokes, gout, and other diseases. Also we can't be sure that it is xanthine oxidase entering the body from homogenized cow's milk which causes our particularly high *American* circulatory disease rate. But this intriguing theory and the extraordinary therapeutic results achieved so far shed a new light on our major killer, heart disease. An important medical breakthrough may be at hand.

This may be especially applicable to young people, for, as we know from autopsy studies of apparently healthy teenagers and young men killed in combat and accidents, severe atherosclerosis now begins at younger and younger ages. This must be dietary in origin because decades of smoking or air pollution have not occurred. Expanded research must now tell us whether the cause is, in fact, this damaging enzyme in homogenized milk. And whether vastly higher levels of folic acid are desirable.

CHAPTER 25:

The Folly of Self-Medication

We have been mentioning many connections between vitamins, nutrition, and human diseases. Some of the connections are close and well known; others are distant or unproved. All together, this may be a bewildering amount of information to the general reader.

Many other books and articles about vitamins have appeared in recent times, some of them enthusiastic and passionate. Many are even urgent, fanatical. It is as if the authors wished to back you up against a wall and hold you there, while they insistently and loudly repeated their message in your ear, so you would be sure to get the point. (If one meets certain health food or vitamin enthusiasts, such may actually happen.)

It is hard to escape the feeling that many of these writers are overselling. They cite example after example. They take quotes from others out of context. They push their arguments far too hard. It is almost as if they cannot help themselves and are forced to exaggerate, even to the extent of hurting their own cause. Their passion seems to drive them to an excess that is self-defeating.

All this sets the alarm bells ringing among physicians, and quite rightly. Sniffing out quackery is a special obligation of medical men. They know that one or two striking cases that cannot be duplicated with other patients does not establish a "cure" for any ailment or condition. They know that unproved notions about easy treatment or cures have cruelly victimized thousands of the gullible and misinformed. They know that vitamins, which are mysterious and potent substances readily available without prescription, have often been used unwisely for self-medication.

The popular writers surely do not wish to deceive. Most vitamin research must be done by dealing with conditions of ill health or disease. There often seems no other way to report the facts about vitamins than by giving the results of these experiments. This tends to stress disease and illness. Indeed, we have too often had to do this ourselves, even though we would have preferred to turn the coin around to the side that signifies good health.

So case after case is cited, and experiment after experiment mentioned, and these are often actual medical or scientific findings. But their number seems excessive, and the results are usually not compared to cases of no result or to other forms of medical treatment for the same illnesses. The reader too easily gets the notion that many or most diseases and disorders of health can be cured by vitamins. This false and dangerous doctrine sets the alarm bells ringing even louder among physicians.

One might wonder why these enthusiasts seem driven by such ardor and zeal. Such strong passions are unlikely to arise merely from the reading of research reports. Why is there such an undercurrent of urgency within many of the new nutritional writings?

Could it be that these passionate crusaders are themselves under healthful nutritional regimens and feel so full of vitality and alertness, such a sense of well-being, that they cannot help sharing their enthusiasm with others? That their own inner feelings of good health are strong enough to drive them compulsively to excess in their opinions and statements, even when this excess is self-defeating?

If so, this would in itself be a sign of the value of vitamin regimens—but their value for health, *not* primarily for the treatment of disease or disorders.

The writers will claim that their statements are all scientifically accurate. Their statements usually are accurate in what they say, but not in what they leave out, the cases where vitamins were not effective, and all the other forms of medical treatments for disease.

The unfortunate implication of many of these writings is that sufferers from a wide range of ailments can get effective relief or be "cured" by vitamins. Then a misguided reader may decide to treat an illness or perhaps attempt an improvement in appearance by using vitamins. Once in a while the consequences are unhappy—perhaps a grossly excessive overdose of vitamin A that will require a doctor's care or hospitalization and will be widely reported in the press.

Or, more commonly, it will happen that a sick person taking vitamins will avoid professional medical guidance and, in the meanwhile, time passes and his condition worsens. Then, much later than he should, he will finally go to a physician. But unnecessary damage will have been caused by the delay.

The ringing of the alarm bells among medical men and women will now rise to a clamor. In fact, many physicians have been turned away from the possible benefits of vitamin regimens by such incidents.

To show the folly of do-it-yourself medicine, let us just consider one example, that of anemia, because many people may have been told, at one time or another, that they are slightly anemic. Usually this anemia is so mild that it poses no real danger to health, so the attending physician made no great fuss about it. But the fact lingers on in the mind of the patient.

Of course, the anemia itself was diagnosed only as a result of a professional blood test, applying modern techniques of medical knowledge. The patient should realize that treatment, if necessary, would also need such expertise.

Anemia is a weakness of the circulating blood, and it can be mild or most severe. It can have many manifestations. There can be too few red blood cells, or these cells can be misshapen, ineffective. Or they may not be sturdy, being instead so fragile that they break open or rupture earlier than they should under normal wear and tear. Or they may contain insufficient hemoglobin, the vital iron-containing pigment that carries oxygen to the cells of the body.

Anemia due to iron deficiency in the diet is not uncommon among a large part of the population, especially among women in the childbearing ages who regularly and normally lose blood by menstruation or who have the extra bodily demands of pregnancy. Generally they cannot get enough iron from their normal food.

But anemia can be due to many nonnutritional causes as well. Infectious diseases can cause anemia. So can many chronic conditions. And anemia can also be hereditary.

Further, anemia may be due to the lack of any one of the following nutrients (in addition to iron): amino acids, vitamins A, B_2, B_6, B_{12}, folic acid, pantothenic acid, PABA, vitamin C, or several minerals (copper, cobalt, zinc, etc.).

So you can see how foolish it would be for anyone with anemia to attempt alone to decide what is its cause and what should be the treatment. Not only are the necessary knowledge and background missing, but so are the important clinical testing and diagnostic procedures to pinpoint the details and monitor the treatment. Even physicians are unlikely to make adequate diagnoses or provide effective treatment without such laboratory tests.

Effective do-it-yourself medicine is thus nearly impossible today, *even for physicians.*

Everybody wants better health and freedom from distressing complaints. In this book, as in others dealing with vitamins and nutrition, we must give examples related to illnesses and health disorders. But these are given to elucidate the properties of vitamins and the functioning of the body and mind, not to suggest that self-medication should be tried. Too often such misguided efforts, however well meaning, can be harmful. Disease may progress to increasingly severe states while do-it-yourself medicine is attempted, without needed diagnostic procedures and without an understanding of the many advances of modern medical knowledge.

Those who try to treat themselves for illnesses or health complaints usually come off far the worse for the effort. Let us repeat that any reader who knows or suspects he is ill, or has a health complaint, should avoid the temptation to doctor himself or herself and should instead see a professional health practitioner.

CHAPTER 26:

The Wisdom of Preventive Medicine

If self-medication for health complaints is foolish and sometimes damaging, there is one area of health care that does properly lie in the province of the layman as well as the doctor.

This is the *prevention* of illness by attaining good health.

Each person's habits and practices are usually mostly his own responsibility, especially his nutritional habits. Although informed medical guidance may be needed to know *what* to do, the "doing" itself rests with the individual: Only he or she can put good principles into practice.

In its broadest sense, preventive medicine comes in many forms. Cleanliness and sterility in the operating room is one way of preventing disease. A quarantine of people or buildings with infectious agents is a preventive practice, as is inoculation with an immunizing vaccine, the killing of disease-carrying insects and rodents, the lowering of pollution levels, and so on.

Good nutrition and the avoidance of life-destroying environments or habits are also important methods of preventive medicine. Perhaps they are the most important, for most of us.

Curing an illness is usually far more dramatic than establishing a preventive procedure. Curative methods are also easier to measure and understand. How can one tell, in the case of an individual patient, why a heart attack, cancer, or a mental breakdown has *not* occurred? One way is to seek indirect links between disease and other factors. For example, Dr. Robert A. Smith and his colleagues at the University of California at Los Angeles raised tissues outside the body from human colon and kidney cancers. They found the cancer cells to have abnormally low concentrations of niacinamide, one form of vitamin B3, establishing such a link.

In a paper published in the *Annals of the New York Academy of Science* entitled "Carcinogenic effects associated with diets deficient in choline and related nutrients," R. W. Engel and others reported on dietary experiments with rats. In one trial, 14 out of 18 rats developed cancers on the choline-deficient diet, while none who received a supplement of 0.2 percent developed such tumors.

Earlier, we have mentioned the cancer-inhibiting properties from other animal experiments of vitamins A, C, and E as well. In a review article in late 1973, the physician Michael B. Shimkin gave some of the early history of cancer research and vitamins:

> Some 35 years ago, Yoshida of Japan reported the appearance of liver cancers in rats maintained on diets to which "butter yellow" and related azo dyes had been added. The news was popularized by Kinosita, who was on a lecture tour in the United States. Practically all our cancer research laboratories existent at that time began to repeat the work. Liver was, and remains, a popular material for biochemical studies. . . .
>
> Surprisingly, rats placed on diets to which azo dyes were added refused to develop liver tumors in the United States. Consultations and investigations soon showed that the key discrepancy between Japan and the United States was in the diet to which the azo dyes were added. In Japan, the rats were maintained on a Spartan diet based on

polished rice. In the United States, the animals were pampered on carefully balanced diets designed for optimum growth. Further investigations pinpointed riboflavin as the main protector against the carcinogenic effects of azo dyes. Rats on riboflavin-deficient diets to which azo dyes were added promptly developed liver tumors as described by Japanese workers.

Much cancer research with vitamins was stimulated by these findings, especially since azo dyes (which do not occur in nature) have been and are widely used as artificial food colorings. Dr. Shimkin again:

Richard S. Rivlin (Columbia University College of Physicians and Surgeons, New York, New York), provides a review on riboflavin and cancer in the September [1973] issue of *Cancer Research*. Rivlin points out that several studies indicate that riboflavin deficiency inhibits tumor growth in experimental animals and possibly in man. There are also provocative observations that certain patients with cancer excrete less riboflavin than do normal individuals. ... The field of vitamin analogues and inhibitors in the treatment of cancer, pioneered by the late Sidney Farber, seems far from exhausted.

Other major baffling diseases are also being linked to vitamins. For example, the Japanese investigator Yakite Ketake and his colleagues have related diabetes to pyridoxine: Using experimental animals, they found that a particular high-fat diet produced diabetic effects, but when pyridoxine was added to this diet, these diabetic manifestations did not appear. Of course, as in so many of these cases, once the disease effects were established, the vitamin could not reverse them.

In addition to such experiments, studies of human population groups (as we have described in the discussion of cardiovascular diseases) are most important to preventive medicine. The point of these studies is to see how disease can be linked to genetic background, dietary habits, patterns of life, or environmental conditions.

Vitamins and Fertility

But disease and ill health conditions are not the only things studied in preventive medicine. Animal experiments are conducted dealing with longevity, rates of growth in the young, fertility, physical size, physical and mental performance, and so on, in order to measure health. Many of these positive factors have been shown to be strongly influenced by nutrition in general and by vitamins in particular.

For example, we know that a separate deficiency of many vitamins or minerals can inhibit or prevent reproduction. Now there is significant new evidence that supplementary choline can add to animal fertility. In 1973 researchers at the University of Missouri reported that additional choline in the diet strongly increased the size of swine litters. Trygve Veum, university researcher, said: "Just adding 1.5 pounds of actual choline per ton of feed increased the number of pigs farrowed and raised to weaning weight by an average of half a pig per litter in our North Central regional research project. Nutritionally speaking, I haven't seen anything that's had such a dramatic effect on litter size in recent years."

It is far too early to draw firm conclusions about human fertility from this finding, but choline is indeed an important, even if often overlooked, vitamin. It is interesting to note that the Food and Nutrition Board stresses choline's protective effects—against poor growth, liver and kidney damage, anemia, muscular weaknesses, cardiovascular diseases, abnormalities in pregnancy and lactation—all of these noted in various animal experiments. (But choline is to be excluded from multivitamin supplements by the new FDA regulations.)

Learning and Intelligence

The positive effects of vitamin intake on human mental functioning is another significant finding. Several vitamins have been found to increase learning and intelligence. For example, in a six-week experiment with 104 children in a Virginia orphanage, as reported in her book *The Effect of Added Thiamin on Learning,* Dr. Ruth Flinn Harrell found that learning ability was improved by about one-fourth by supplemental thiamin. Physical skills were also improved. The benefits applied to both normal and retarded children.

Before the trial there were no signs of thiamin deficiency, but the experiment shows that formerly the children were obviously not receiving enough thiamin for optimal performance.

Vitamin C has similarly been shown to improve intelligence by psychologists A. L. Kubala and M. M. Katz, who did experiments in three cities with 351 students ranging in age from kindergarten to college. The students were first tested by means of blood samples for existing vitamin C levels, and then given IQ tests. In each of the four schools involved, there were higher average IQ's at the beginning among the students who had normally higher vitamin C levels.

Then additional orange juice was given to all. There was an across-the-board IQ increase, but it was slight among the preexisting high vitamin C-high IQ group, and substantial among those who began with lower vitamin and lower IQ levels.

Vitamins and Old Age

Longevity is another way to measure health. We know that there is a great variation in life span, both among individuals and between different societies. In our own culture, painters and philosophers, poets and scientists, artists, judges, musicians, and statesmen have often led fruitful and creative lives into their eighties and beyond.

Titian was still painting when he succumbed to the plague at 99, Pablo Picasso signed his last canvas over 90, and Grandma Moses painted into her one hundred and first year. The poet Conrad Aiken said: "It's refreshing to be discovered even at the age of eighty," and published his last poem at 83. Bertrand Russell's final book appeared when he was 91, Churchill resigned his leadership at 80, DeGaulle at 78, but Justice Oliver Wendell Holmes continued working at 90. Many scientists have also worked happily and productively into a ripe old age of contentment, activity, and achievement.

Never before have the secrets of aging—and of *not* aging—been so deeply investigated as in our own time. The goal is not just long life, but active and healthful later years. Dr. Christopher Cook of the Association of Life Insurance Medical Directors, and a particular vitamin E enthusiast, has noted that the medical meaning of aging is not wisdom and serenity. "Aging in medicine means deterioration. It means a slower gait, dimmer eyesight, harder breathing, shakier hands, less and less enjoyment of all the pleasures—food, talk, laughter, love, sex, sleeping, getting up, social interest, using one's brain—of life."

High-level intakes of vitamin E, according to Dr. Cook, can do much to delay or minimize these unwelcome states, and thus delay medical aging.

Further, let us again note the belief of Dr. Abram Hoffer, the pioneer in schizophrenia treatment by orthomolecular methods, that senility is not inevitable, but is most often due to long-term nutritional deficiencies.

Animal experiments are beginning to relate vitamins more directly to longevity. For example, the B vitamin pantothenic acid (also taken in the form calcium pantothenate) is an important constituent of royal jelly. This is the dietary substance that keeps honey bee embryos from becoming short-lived infertile workers, and makes them instead develop into the queen bee, who is very long-lived and very fertile.

In one experiment, one group of mice was fed a standard diet, while a second and similar group received the same diet, but with supplemental pantothenic acid added. The mice in the first group lived an average of 550 days. Those in the second outlived them by an average of 103 days. This is an increase of nearly 20 percent, highly significant statistically. Such a great increase in longevity deserves many follow-up studies because the possibilities of human benefit are profound.

Most investigators who have specialized in aging and longevity have become convinced of the primary importance of nutrition and exercise to youthful later years of life, with the wisdom and serenity that age should bring, but without the physical or mental deterioration that all too often now occur. Such long-term health must be the aim of preventive medical practices.

The chronic and degenerative complaints that are the major health problems of our time also affect the elderly with special force. Many of these ailments arise from decades of exposure to environmental hazards, of bad health habits, and of unwise dietary practices. Seeking "cures" for these ailments has not been noticeably successful and at best can only be a stopgap measure. We must learn to prevent these diseases before they start.

The Importance of Preventive Medicine

A higher medical status and additional respect are now coming to preventive medicine, as this point of view becomes more widely realized. Two new professional journals, for example, were begun in 1972, *Preventive Medicine* in the United States and *Prevent* in Great Britain, to join existing periodicals, such as the *Journal of the International Academy of Preventive Medicine*.

Organized professional leadership is necessary if the findings of preventive medicine are to come out of the laboratory and research studies and be realized in the form of better health and greater longevity for all.

Providing such leadership are the long-established Academy of Applied Nutrition and Association of Family Physicians, the newer International Academy of Preventive Medicine and American Health Foundation, and the very recently formed Academy of Orthomolecular Psychiatry (which held its first national meeting in 1972), geriatric and gerontological groups, and other professional associations.

These organizations stress a renewed concern for the *whole entity* that is any human being. Once a characteristic of medicine in the old horse-and-buggy days when the family physician knew all aspects of his patients intimately, much of this disappeared in the rush toward specialization in the late 1940's. Happily, such a holistic concern for the health as well as the illnesses of their patients is now beginning to return among many responsible physicians.

But preventive medicine is not wholly in the hands of the doctors. More than any other health practice, it is the personal responsibility of every individual who wishes to live a satisfying and healthful existence. Nutrition —especially the vitamin, mineral, and protein plans we have described earlier—should be everybody's concern.

CHAPTER 27:

The FDA and the Risk
of National Malnutrition

> Vitamins and minerals are supplied in abundant amounts by commonly available foods. Except for persons with special medical needs, there is no scientific basis for recommending routine use of dietary supplements.

This statement has been proposed by the Food and Drug Administration to be placed prominently on the label of every vitamin product.

It is "inaccurate and misleading," commented Assistant Secretary of Agriculture George L. Mehren, who pointed out it would give a consumer who was eating unwisely "a false sense of security." "The statement is not true," flatly stated the distinguished scientist Linus Pauling. It is a proposal of "no relevance . . . which taken out of context creates a false impression," said Dr. William H. Sebrell, chairman of the Committee on Recommended Dietary Allowances of the National Academy of Sciences, National Research Council.

Such criticism of the Food and Drug Administration's approach to vitamins has come from every side over the past decade and continues to grow steadily.

For example, the CBS news program *60 Minutes* often contains a segment entitled "Point Counterpoint" in which two famed newspaper columnists from opposite ends of the political spectrum offer comments on the hap-

330 The Doctor's Book on Vitamin Therapy

penings of the world. Representing the left is witty, sar-
castic, irreverent Nicholas von Hoffman. In 1973 he wrote
that those who oppose the FDA's vitamin regulations,

> . . . will dispute them with a fury born of a desire to live
> long and healthy lives. When these same people recall the
> ignorance of the physicians who fail at ministering to
> them, they react with something like rage when the FDA
> declares, "Lay persons are incapable of determining by
> themselves whether they have, or are likely to develop,
> vitamin or mineral deficiencies."
>
> A generation ago people were cowed by such assertions
> . . . by the alliance of government power and medicine,
> but now too many doctors have killed too many patients
> with too many dangerous drugs for well-informed people
> to accept such claims. Our mortality rates are too high and
> our level of health care too low and people know it.
>
> The FDA has mounted a campaign that suggests anyone
> who opposes it, the medical cartels, and the drug com-
> panies, are kooks, faddists, and secret sympathizers with
> the John Birch Society. People once thought much the
> same of Pasteur, for it has been the peculiar tradition of
> medicine in the last 200 or 300 years to prefer exorcism
> and excommunication of new hypotheses to the scientific
> testing of them.
>
> The non-MDs and even some of the doctors will not be
> intimidated by old dogmas and old dogmatists even if they
> are enforced by the power of the state. . . .

As if not to be outdone, the astute conservative colum-
nist James J. Kilpatrick, the opposite side of CBS's "Point
Counterpoint," also wrote bitingly about the FDA's vitamin statements and proposals:

> What is most irritating in all this—and in a profoundly
> disturbing way most ominous—is the commissioner's will-
> ingness to lay down, as a matter of law, what is "scientifi-
> cally accurate." He establishes certain U.S. Recom-
> mended Daily Allowances for Vitamins and Minerals and

declares it "scientifically correct" that products be so labeled. He rules it "scientifically inaccurate" to list a dietary property "that is of no significance in human nutrition." It is "scientifically inaccurate" to make certain statements about "the quality of the soil in the United States."

When the federal government begins writing into law what is scientifically accurate, it is later than we think. Most of us had supposed that such monumental folly had vanished even from the Soviet Union. When mere expert opinions and prestigious recommendations are converted into binding regulations—not to protect the public safety but merely to relieve consumer confusion—government oversteps its bounds.

The FDA's newest proposed regulations, announced in 1973, were accompanied by a listing of so-called "Findings of Fact," several of which are not only nonfactual (being merely opinions) but actually false or self-contradictory. For example,

> There is no relationship between the vitamin content of foods and the chemical composition of the soil in which they are grown.

False. It is well known that proper soil content does indeed relate to the vitamins in the plants grown on it. Suitable chemical fertilizers, in particular, can do much to boost the vitamin content. A. Voisin's 1959 book *Soil, Grass and Cancer,* for example, describes how fertilization with nitrogen-potash-phosphate substantially increased the provitamin-A content of plants over fertilization with manure only. Other experiments have shown that similar fertilization has doubled the Vitamin B_1 content of grains. It is only common sense to know that fertile soils produce plants with higher nutrient content.

> Mineral nutrients in food are not significantly affected by storage, transportation, cooking, and other processing.

False. The minerals in wheat and sugarcane (or sugar beets) are largely removed when the plants are processed into white patent flour and refined sugar. Nearly all of the calcium, magnesium, etc., are removed. Also, when minerals are present in foods in the form of water-soluble salts, as often happens, vegetables cooked in water can lose much of their mineral content into the cooking water.

The term "subclinical" and similar ill-defined terms when used to define vitamin and mineral deficiencies . . . are neither informative nor meaningful to consumers. . . .

False and self-contradictory. The FDA claims to draw its scientific knowledge primarily from the work of the Food and Nutrition Board and states that this Board's 1968 report, *Recommended Dietary Allowances (Seventh Revised Edition),* "should be used as the source of authentic and reliable information" about nutritional matters. But this report does state, in dealing with a particular nutrient (linoleic acid, one of the essential fatty acids), that in some cases supplements may be necessary "to prevent a *subclinical* physiologic deficiency . . . " (page 12, emphasis added). About pantothenic acid, the report states (page 39), "biochemical defects may exist undetected for a time . . ." which is the meaning of "subclinical." (Let us also recall the long time period during which Dr. Fitch's vitamin E-deprived monkeys demonstrated no overt sign of deficiency; the admitted marginal or lacking iron stores among many women which produce no immediate clinical signs; etc.)

The Food and Nutrition Board's report also refers in this vein to magnesium (page 60, emphasis added): "Animals fed moderately low levels of magnesium, *sufficient to allow normal growth and prevent all gross signs of deficiency,* often develop calcified lesions of the soft tissues and increased susceptibility to the atherogenic effects of cholesterol feeding. . . ." That is, severely damaging magnesium deficiencies in animals may also be "subclinical."

Such erroneous "Findings of Fact" have led many to suspect the fervor with which the FDA has approached the vitamin field. The FDA's vitamin hearings have dragged on for a decade, cost hundreds of thousands of dollars, produced 26,000 pages of testimony—all designed to prove that vitamin supplements are unnecessary. "This position has been increasingly embarrassing for the agency," notes James S. Turner's *The Chemical Feast* (The Ralph Nader Study Group Report). "The FDA found itself opposing vitamin supplementation just at a time when vitamin deficiencies were becoming a major national concern. Scientists and researchers in the field of nutrition have been appalled by the FDA's activities in the vitamin field almost since they began."

The FDA's proposed new vitamin regulations, described earlier, have drawn much severe criticism from many sources, including Republican Congressman Craig Hosmer of California, who commented:

What the Food and Drug Administration seeks to do is to classify foods, food supplements, concentrated foods, and vitamin and mineral products as drugs. It would effectively do so by imposing an arbitrary limit on the quantity of any vitamin or mineral which may be used in a single tablet or capsule, whether or not the product is established as harmful in larger doses.

But, as any biomedical scientist can tell you, there are basic differences between nutrients and typical drugs.

• Nutrients furnish the building blocks for construction of the body's enzyme systems that make metabolism possible. Drugs do not do so. Thus, if a substance acts constructively, it must be a nutrient, not a drug.

• Nutrients act like a team within the body, but drugs act individually by interfering with metabolism processes.

• Typically, nutrients are native to the body, while drugs in general are foreign, alien substances.

The absurdity of defining vitamins in terms of something they are not was pointed out by the famed scientist Linus Pauling when he noted:

"If the proposed limitation of the sale of Vitamin A were extended to foods, a prescription would be required for a serving of one half of one ounce of broiled lamb liver or two ounces of sweet potatoes. The FDA is either wrong in proposing the limitation on the sale of capsules . . . or remiss in not also proposing the equivalent limitation on the sale of liver, sweet potatoes, and other foods. . . ."

The inconsistency of FDA's double standard is also clearly manifested in its truthful but misleading claim that *"at this time"* no vitamin or mineral will be removed from the shelves or restricted to solely prescription use.

You can't have it both ways.

If certain vitamins are proven to be so harmful that they must be taken under a physician's guidance, then they are dangerous enough to be prescribed. If they are not put under prescription, then this becomes another meaningless, unenforceable regulation, likely to become institutionalized as one more area in which the consumers are denied freedom to think for themselves. . . .

The consumer is not an irrational imbecile who needs his life programmed by commercialism's money interest or bureaucracy's penchant for running other people's lives . . . Laws already on the books give FDA adequate authority to protect the consumer against dosages which may be harmful if excessive. In cases where there is no indication of this result—any more than from intaking inordinate amounts of water—no new laws or regulations are necessary to protect the consumer against large dosages which are not known to be harmful.

After all, FDA's Recommended Daily Allowances are only the product of man. They were not carved on a mountain in stone. It just may be that the intake of a harmless nutrient or vitamin actually does improve some people's well-being. . . .

To support these views, Representative Hosmer has introduced legislation (H.R. 643) to overturn the FDA's proposed regulations. Similarly, Senator William Proxmire (Democrat, Wisconsin) has proposed a bill, S. 2801, in the Senate to halt the FDA from putting its regulations into effect in 1975. Senator Proxmire's bill has gathered 38 cosponsors, including many political luminaries such as Senators Barry Goldwater, Hubert Humphrey, George McGovern, and the Democratic and Republican leaders, Mike Mansfield and Hugh Scott. From Southerners (Eastland, Talmadge, Sparkman, etc.) to Northerners (Pell, Schweiker, etc.) to Midwesterners and Texans (Dole, Tower, Bensten) to Far-Westerners (Tunney, Gravel, Hatfield), Senators of every political persuasion have joined to cosponsor this important legislation.

Readers of this book whose own well-being and health are benefited by our proposed vitamin regimens may have a greater stake in this controversy than the average citizen. One way to express this is to write to the FDA Commissioner: Dr. A. M. Schmidt, Commissioner, Food and Drug Administration, 5600 Fishers Lane, Rockville, Maryland 20852. Or perhaps more effectively, one can write to his or her Congressman, Senator, or the President. *Request their support of the Hosmer and Proxmire bills, H.R. 643 and S. 2801, to overturn the FDA's foolish regulations.* Your letters or cards can be addressed to:

The Honorable . . .
U.S. House of Representatives
Washington, D.C. 20515

The Honorable . . .
U.S. Senate
Washington, D.C. 20510

The President of the United States
The White House
Washington, D.C. 20500

Faults of the FDA

Why has the FDA adopted such an anti-vitamin stance? Some critics point to the relationship of FDA officials to big business, especially the large pharmaceutical companies, who may stand to gain greatly from these regulations, as we shall see.

Instances of outright corruption in other areas within the FDA have indeed come to light. In one case, the FDA diluted warnings about the health dangers of birth control pills, which came up in court testimony when one victim suffered brain damage as a result. Physicians were not given sufficient information by the watered-down birth control pill warning, said Dr. Robert S. McCleery, who had earlier resigned from the FDA "to protest the timidity and foot-dragging of the FDA's top echelon in stopping the sale of combinations of antibiotics that had been found unsafe," according to the Washington *Post*.

In another instance, an attorney departing from the FDA provided his new employer with the confidential details of the FDA file on the company and on a forthcoming legal case. The uproar over this disclosure cost the attorney his new job and embarrassed all concerned.

Of course there are rascally federal bureaucrats, just as there are rascally doctors and priests. In the case of the FDA, because life-and-death matters are often involved, special vigilance is surely needed. But a greater concern for the welfare of business than the health and welfare of the public has seemed to characterize many FDA decisions of policy.

The most recent controversy came after the FDA announced in 1973 that hereafter it will no longer inform the public (or physicians) about dangerous situations that require recalling from the market of foods, drugs, or medical devices. Hitherto, such recalls to protect the public health were openly announced. Now they will be kept confidential. The reason cited is that the public might be unduly alarmed by such announcements. For example, the wearer of a heart pacemaker (an electronic device inserted in the body to provide needed electrical stimulation to the heart) might read in his morning newspaper that his pacemaker model is defective and then suffer a heart attack from fright!

Many unhappy reactions greeted this news announcement. "Irresponsible and indefensible ... the height of arrogance," said Dr. Sidney Wolfe. "This policy is in the best interests of the medical device, drug, and food industries, but in the worst interests of the patients, other consumers, and doctors who more than likely will suffer from not having been informed about these problems."

Another commentator summed up the case against the FDA: "A government agency wants to resolve the problem by arbitrarily deciding each case devoid of public scrutiny. In a democratic society—which at least purports to subscribe to the ideal of a free flow of information—such a policy is unsatisfactory."

As in its vitamin policy, again the FDA seems to be selling the public short, to the benefit of the large food and drug companies from which many of its staff members come and in which many of them will later find employment.

By stirring up the vitamin situation, certain to draw tens of thousands of letters from the public and much notice in Congress, the FDA will have its poor record overlooked in dealing with drugs, damaging food additives, pesticides, and consumer fraud by mislabeling and mispackaging. Among those pointing this out is the Nader Study Group, whose report asserts that "eliminating the vitamin hearings would free badly needed resources" to cope with more important matters, and the record on vitamins is "an almost incredible sample of FDA bungling. . . . The FDA's mishandling of the vitamin hearings is unusual in that it alienated both the consuming public and a segment of the food industry [that now manufactures vitamins]."

Favoring Big Business

Today, dozens and dozens of small companies manufacture and sell vitamin products. Though the large pharmaceutical supercorporations often also produce vitamins, this is only a small part of their total business. Vitamins are free and unpatentable compounds, open to manufacture by all. The pharmaceutical giants prefer drugs that they can sell exclusively, as is the case with many antibiotics, tranquilizers, etc. With these, they can get high prices and be legally protected by patents against competition.

If the new FDA regulations are allowed to stand, then high-level vitamin capsules and tablets (over 150 percent of the U.S. RDA) will be classified as "drugs." In order that a company sell a drug, it must be proved that it is both *efficacious* and *safe,* or, at least, relatively safe. Testing, especially for efficacy, is often expensive and time-consuming—beyond the resources of most small companies.

The new regulations would then give several advantages to the large drug giants. They, and not their small competitors, can afford to test disputed vitamins (perhaps in new chemical forms that can be patented), while the small companies may be forbidden from selling them at all. This could apply to PABA, inositol, etc. The better known and undisputed vitamins may also have to have a proof of efficacy and safety before large-dose tablets and capsules can be sold; here, too, the larger companies will have the advantage. They can test and prove efficacy (again, possibly in patentable forms), and then proceed to sell almost the same vitamins to the public, while the smaller companies could not keep up because these will be called *drugs.*

Further, the single type of multivitamin *supplement* to become standard means that individual distinctions among different vitamin products will tend to disappear. Many small companies now sell individualistic mixtures of vitamins in varying potencies. Some of these mixtures certainly are foolish and irrational, but many are desirable. If the law only permits a single type of vitamin supplement, it is far easier for one or two giant companies, skilled in advertising and with large budgets, to advertise incessantly and capture the bulk of the market—as has happened with so many food products.

All of the above can happen, even *if prescriptions are never required for most vitamins.* If, in addition, prescriptions become necessary for 500-mg vitamin C pills, for example, the large pharmaceutical companies will have a greater advantage. They have the best arrangements with drug wholesalers and pharmacists and can provide prescription products at lower (wholesale) prices. The small companies could be squeezed out altogether.

If the reader senses a contradiction, he is judging too quickly. We have earlier approved of two principles in the proposed FDA regulations: that vitamins and minerals, if present in a supplement, should be there in meaningful quantities, and all the essential vitamins should be present. This much is to the good. Most of the rest is to the bad.

A more fruitful regulation would have been to require that *if a known nutrient is present and advertised, it should be so in a meaningful quantity, and all multipurpose or one-a-day pills should have all the known essential vitamins.* Also, all extraneous fillers, bindings, and coatings should be listed on vitamin labels, for it is thought that these may be the real cause of "vitamin" side effects (rashes, gastric upsets, etc.), not the vitamins themselves.

This much—and no more—would protect the public against deception and fraud, permit the smaller companies to continue their competition, and improve the quality of many vitamin and mineral supplements. It would also allow those who know they benefit from higher vitamin intakes than 150 percent of the U.S. RDA to continue to buy those supplements without fearing that these will be withdrawn from the market. And those who wish to take the disputed vitamins (and possibly trace nutrients in desiccated liver, wheat germ powder, etc.) can have that benefit, too.

As they stand, the proposed regulations will give a major business advantage to the giant "ethical" drug companies. Vitamin prices will probably rise. And, more seriously, many persons unwilling or unable to get a physician's prescription for vitamins, may even have to forgo their needed vitamins.

Promoting National Malnutrition

The Food and Drug Administration itself proclaims that its 1973 proposed U.S. RDA's and vitamin-mineral supplement regulations should be sufficient for nearly all "normally healthy" persons—95 to 99 percent of them, it claims.

At first glance, this looks adequate. But without wishing to split hairs finely or quarrel unduly, let us take this statement at face value and look closely at the figures. Our total population is well over 200,000,000, and we know that 11 percent, or at least 22,000,000 human beings, are unfortunately chronically ill to some degree. At any given time another approximately 10,000,000 persons are sick or injured—suffering from colds or other minor illnesses, broken limbs, serious infections, recuperating from surgery, and so on. Added together, this gives a total of about 32,000,000 or more, leaving roughly 170,000,000 of the "normally healthy." Suppose there actually are 5 percent of these, or 8.5 million persons, for whom the U.S. RDA's are insufficient.

Add it all up and there could be some *40,000,000 Americans* for whom the U.S. RDA's—and the vitamin supplement limitations based on them—would be insufficient. We draw this deduction from the FDA's and Food and Nutrition Board's own evaluation of their vitamin and mineral allowances.

For the population as a whole, then, the proposed new

regulations would then impose a *20 percent or greater risk of malnutrition.* It seems to us this is an unwise and potentially dangerous public health risk. And a totally unnecessary one. Why should it exist? To spare the public some occasional slight unneeded vitamin expenditures? To increase the prosperity of already very profitable large pharmaceutical companies? Why should we so risk malnutrition and associated disease on such a vast national scale when our public health is already in decline?

CHAPTER 28:

A Doctor's Hope

It is the business of physicians to deal daily with sickness and injury, pain and suffering. This is often demanding work, both physically and at the deepest levels of the human spirit.

Medical history is illuminated by many heroic examples, even in nutritional research. Dr. Joseph Goldberger, for example, faced skepticism in his claims that pellagra was not a contagious disease. To prove his point, he injected nasal mucus, scale, and even excrement into his own body, and those of his associates and his wife, thereby advancing our knowledge of this mortal vitamin deficiency.

But the average doctor and other health professional, who would not be called heroic or think of himself or herself that way, may also confront serious disease and pain among his or her patients. (It is for good reason that doctors themselves have a high incidence of alcoholism, drug addiction, mental breakdown, and shortened lives. The demands and strain of the work can be extreme.)

And even though health professionals try to alleviate and avoid pain, it is a most valuable part of human functioning. Our race would not have survived long without it. Pain tells us something has gone amiss in our bodies and needs rapid attention.

Similarly, though more often overlooked, depression can be a valuable state. Depression means a person has somehow gone awry—whether this be in job or career, personal or family life, diet and nutrition, or bodily, via a disease-related cause, such as a bacterial or viral infection, or a degenerative disorder.

All such signs and symptoms are important clues to treatment. As medical science continues to advance, more fine details and knowledge continue to emerge, and we can hope to be more successful in understanding the causes of our physical and behavioral maladies and in treating them. Most significant, we are learning that many of our health complaints are unnecessary, preventable in advance.

As we have tried to describe in this book, vitamins and nutrition are today seeing a great upsurge in medical interest. These will be increasingly important, we predict, in the medicine of the future.

But there are certain related problems that transcend matters of individual health, problems in which nutrition has had a major—though often hidden or overlooked—role. Burning social and political issues may be at stake.

Race, Poverty, and Malnutrition

No domestic problem has caused more bitterness or been so destructive in our society than the race problem. Investigators with much education in sociology or psychology—but little in biomedical matters and nutrition—have examined one or another aspect of racial prejudices and differences, but unfortunately, many of them have lacked the knowledge to understand their own findings.

So-called intelligence (IQ) testing has been very popular in recent years. Apparently, it has been easy to get research funds for such paper-and-pencil studies among population groups, because we have had an abundance of them. Easier still is to "interpret" the studies of others. Very little of this work has been useful, and much has been meaningless. But some of it, including the most publicized, has been of surpassing foolishness. Often it has been conducted (or commented upon) by nutritional ignoramuses, regardless of their degrees or status in other fields.

One study, for example, led to the impressive findings that poor people have less money than other groups, greater rates of crime and personal instability, and weaker family structures. Further, the impoverished score lower on intelligence tests. Of course, included among the poverty-stricken are proportionately greater numbers of black Americans and those in other minority groups.

In particular, black Americans have not statistically matched their white counterparts (or members of some other minority groups) in school performance and on IQ tests. The poorer performance by blacks is ascribed in whole or part to inherited and unchangeable factors. Some psychologists, led by Arthur Jensen and others, conclude that there are basic mental differences between these groups. William Shockley, a Nobel Prize-winning physicist (for research in transistors), has also been a leader in expounding this point of view. One would like to think that nutritional ignorance, rather than malice, lies behind these erroneous views.

Jensen, Shockley, and their followers would have us believe that blacks are inherently less intelligent than whites, and also less intelligent than Orientals and American Indians. This is supposed to be a fundamental genetic inferiority of people of African descent.

But it is far more likely, as former U.S. Attorney General Ramsey Clark points out in his perceptive book *Crime in America*, that poor nutrition and home environments are the root causes of all such lower performance.

Dozens and dozens of studies tell us, for example, that the nutrition of the mother-to-be affects her unborn child. Not only general good or bad nutrition, but even seasonal variations in nutrition are believed to have psychological effects, based on dietary changes.

Dr. Hare and Dr. Price, for example, classified the birth month of all patients admitted to Bethlem-Maudsley Hospital in London over a 12-year period, from 1951 to 1963. There were more neurotic patients resulting from spring births, when there are also more births in the population at large, but more schizophrenics were born in the winter quarter. They could not pinpoint a reason but speculated that protein deficiencies in the mothers' summer diets, or vitamin C deficiencies in children born in the winter, might be related.

Not only prenatal nutrition, but also nutrition during the early years of infancy and childhood can have lifelong effect on intelligence, temperament, and personality, as well as on physical growth and general health.

The impoverished groups at the bottom of the socioeconomic ladder tend to be the least well nourished *in ways that are most likely to affect the unborn child and growing infant.* In particular, the lack of abundant proteins, vitamin-rich foods, and sufficient minerals can have the most effect.

The hamburger-fries-Coke diet of the middle-class teen-ager and the two-Martini-steak-dab-of-salad repast of the executive may represent types of poor nutrition common among the affluent, but these are not likely to affect the next generation. Middle class and wealthy mothers are also often malnourished, but many types of their malnutrition are different *in kind* from those among the poor.

Among the affluent we often find "overnutrition"—the vitamins and minerals are usually there, but swamped in the expectant mother's metabolism by the "empty calories" that surround them. The developing fetus can still usually (though not always) extract enough nutrients for his own needs, which may not be the case in the diets of the poor where the expectant mothers may be deprived in a more absolute sense.

We are only at the beginnings of our knowledge of molecular biology and cellular nutrition. The various ethnic groups—blacks, American Indians, Orientals—also have *different idiosyncratic typical diets.* These may contain subtle nutritional differences whose effects could be especially pronounced at the beginning of life, during the prenatal, infant, and childhood periods. Then their influence will carry forward throughout a lifetime.

Senator Ernest Hollings, formerly governor of South Carolina, testified poignantly and sensibly on this point before the U.S. Senate Select Committee on Nutrition and Human Needs:

> The reason hardly any of the hungry are designated as "starving" is that our society will take the ill in his last stages and get him to a hospital for treatment. For the $65 a day there—and that is what it costs at the hospital, what the costs are in Charleston [1969]—we could feed an entire hungry family for a week . . . The Committee must learn that it is cheaper to feed the child than jail the man.
>
> Now the medical facts need emphasizing. Dr. Charles Lowe has just testified a few weeks ago before the committee that the brain cells of the human being form during the first 4 years. *Because of the lack of nutrition there is often as much as a 20-percent loss in the brain cell development.* [Emphasis added.]

Nutrition, not genetic differences, is probably the cause of the reported IQ differences between the races. By all the valid scientific evidence, in the light of both our nutritional knowledge and our nutritional ignorance, the studies purporting to show there are inherited unchangeable differences in intelligence among the human races must be considered rubbish.

Because of the manner of development of the human nervous system, we must try to prevent mental impairment (and attain maximum performance) by adequate nutrition at the right time, so we are not forced to repair the damage after it is done. In some cases the damage is tragically irreversible.

Toward a Better National and Personal Health

We are a malnutritious nation. Our health has been corrupted by the big food and drug companies and by the modern practices of agricultural and other businesses. Our own personal habits are also working against us, whether these be our eating habits or our compulsion to drive polluting automobiles instead of walking or bicycling the short distances that most of our trips require.

As we continue to misuse our bodies (and minds), the situation worsens. National and personal health decline. Aberrations occur in the political and moral spheres, as well as those that can be measured in the form of hospital admissions, needless early deaths, and chronic, debilitating illnesses. A mental malaise is widespread, as the joy and spontaneity of good health seem to elude us.

A *national health program* is urgently needed. Without it we will decline further as a nation and a society. This program must seek first, on a nearly emergency basis, to benefit the elderly who are often beset by long illnesses with soaring costs they cannot afford. "Almost every elderly person has arthritis or trouble walking or is short of breath or has something wrong," notes Dr. Helen Hackman, director of Virginia's Arlington County Department of Human Resources, who commented that essential yet comparatively simple requirements such as out-of-hospital medications, hearing aids, eyeglasses, or dental work are often not readily provided under existing medical care programs.

Also, "sometimes there's a situation where malnutrition is not due to just a lack of proper diet, but to a lack of money to buy dentures to eat the food."

Proper nutritional supplements, especially of vitamins and minerals, must also be provided to those whose health is in sore need of them.

Our government agencies, especially the Food and Drug Administration, but also the U.S. Department of Agriculture, must begin to put the welfare of the public above the profits of the large corporations they all too often serve.

Special attention must be devoted to children, or we will perpetuate a bad health situation for another generation. This includes a revision of our thinking about prenatal care. We now have far too many excessively nervous, hyperactive children thronging our medical clinics because their mothers became malnourished when treated with diuretics and amphetamines to lose weight during their pregnancies. These drugged mothers may have given us a whole generation of children who tend toward serious allergies and will have other severe chemoneurological signs.

The removal of damaging artificial food additives, more stringent controls over pollutants and fertilizers, and an end to the chemical distortion of our farm livestock, would all be valuable steps toward improving the nation's health. A greater supply of vitamins and minerals in fresh wholesome food would pay for itself many times over in hospital bills and medical and dental care, not to mention human suffering and longevity.

A *personal health program* for every individual is also needed. Exercise suitable to one's physical condition, sufficient sleep and recreation, and above all, good nutrition, are the key elements in such a program. The vitamin and mineral supplements that we have proposed can be most important.

The newer Health Maintenance Organizations, called HMO's, offer a fairly complete program of health care to families fortunate enough to be in the right locality and be accepted for membership. For a flat monthly fee, all members of the family can have most of their health needs attended to by knowledgeable professionals, including surgery and other forms of treatment that otherwise might be financially crushing.

But paid-up "crisis care" is not the whole answer, neither in a national nor in a personal health program.

Such care only deals with that which should be preventable. Neglect often exacts a high price—in money, in time, and in suffering. HMO's and national health systems will have their highest merit if they establish wise preventive programs, including restorative vitamin regimens, to help overcome so many disorders before they start and to build better disease-resisting health among all of us.

One commentator on our total health picture, as quoted in the New York *Times,* movingly expressed the thrust of this promising new medical attitude: "It is not enough to pay sentimental tribute to the ideal family doctor, the 'Marcus Welby's' of television make-believe and public yearning. . . .

"We must now create the institutions and conditions to make it possible for real live doctors to be both scientists and humanists, and to shift their primary attitudes from crisis intervention to lifetime prevention and health maintenance."

This, it may be said, could be a doctor's hope. Boosting health rather than treating illness.